DR. NOW'S

1200-CALORIE DIET PLAN

Unlock Dr. Nowzaradan's Proven Formula for Rapid Weight Loss and Lasting Health with Quick, Easy, and Delicious Recipes. Includes Expert Tips and a 120-Day Meal Plan.

Rosalind J Hale

Table of Contents

INTRODUCTION

OVERVIEW OF DR. NOWZARADAN'S DIET PRINCIPLES

Dr. Younan Nowzaradan, often referred to as Dr. Now, has gained widespread recognition for his unique approach to weight loss, particularly through his work on the reality television series "My 600-lb Life." His diet principles are centered around a 1200-calorie-per-day regimen, designed to initiate rapid weight loss in individuals who are severely obese, preparing them for bariatric surgery. This diet is not just about limiting calorie intake but is structured around a high-protein, low-carbohydrate, and low-fat framework. The primary goal is to ensure that the body receives adequate nutrition—vitamins, minerals, and protein—while significantly reducing calorie consumption to promote weight loss.

The foundation of Dr. Nowzaradan's diet is to create a calorie deficit, meaning the body uses more calories for energy than it receives from food, thus forcing it to burn stored fat for energy. This principle is crucial for individuals with a significantly high body mass index (BMI), as it can lead to immediate health improvements and reduce the risk of developing obesity-related complications. The high-protein aspect of the diet helps in preserving muscle mass during the weight loss process, which is essential for maintaining a healthy metabolism. Low carbohydrate intake helps in reducing insulin levels and aids in the reduction of stored fat. Meanwhile, keeping fat intake low ensures that calorie consumption is controlled, as fats are more calorie-dense than proteins or carbohydrates.

Dr. Nowzaradan's diet principles also emphasize the importance of portion control and making informed food choices. Processed and high-sugar foods are discouraged, while vegetables, lean meats, and whole grains are recommended. Understanding and implementing these dietary principles can be a challenge, especially for individuals who are used to consuming much higher amounts of calories. However, the structured approach, when followed diligently, can lead to significant weight loss and health improvements, making it a powerful tool in the fight against obesity.

BENEFITS OF THE DR. NOWZARADAN DIET

Adhering to the Dr. Nowzaradan diet offers a multitude of benefits that extend beyond mere weight loss. This diet, structured around a 1200-calorie daily intake, emphasizes high-protein, low-carbohydrate, and low-fat foods, which collectively contribute to a healthier lifestyle. One of the primary advantages is the promotion of rapid weight loss, which is crucial for individuals facing severe obesity. This swift reduction in weight can significantly decrease the risk of obesity-related health issues, such as diabetes, hypertension, and heart disease, thereby improving overall health and longevity.

The high protein content of the diet aids in preserving muscle mass during the weight loss process. Maintaining muscle is essential not only for strength and mobility but also because muscle tissue burns more calories at rest compared to fat tissue, thus enhancing metabolic rate. This can lead to more sustainable weight management in the long term.

Furthermore, the diet's low carbohydrate approach helps in stabilizing blood sugar levels, which can reduce cravings and minimize the likelihood of insulin resistance. This is particularly beneficial for individuals with type 2 diabetes or those at risk of developing this condition. By focusing on low-fat foods, the diet also encourages the consumption of healthier fat sources, which can support heart health and reduce cholesterol levels.

Another significant benefit is the emphasis on whole foods and the exclusion of processed items, which not only aids in weight loss but also ensures that the body is nourished with essential vitamins, minerals, and fiber. This can lead to improved digestion, increased energy levels, and better overall well-being.

Lastly, following the Dr. Nowzaradan diet can empower individuals with the knowledge and habits necessary for making healthier food choices. This education and experience can instill a lifelong commitment to maintaining a healthy weight and lifestyle, ultimately leading to a higher quality of life.

CHAPTER 1: UNDERSTANDING THE DR. NOWZARADAN DIET

1.1: THE SCIENCE BEHIND THE DIET

1.1.1: Low-Calorie, High-Protein Principles

The low-calorie, high-protein, low-fat principles form the cornerstone of Dr. Nowzaradan's diet plan, designed to promote weight loss while ensuring the body receives essential nutrients. This dietary approach focuses on reducing calorie intake to create a calorie deficit, which is fundamental for weight loss. By consuming fewer calories than the body expends, it begins to use stored fat for energy, leading to weight loss.

High-protein foods play a critical role in this diet for several reasons. First, protein is more satiating than carbohydrates or fats, which helps reduce overall calorie intake by keeping hunger at bay between meals. This makes it easier for individuals to adhere to a low-calorie diet without experiencing constant hunger. Second, protein has a higher thermic effect than other macronutrients, meaning the body uses more energy to digest and metabolize it. This increases the overall calorie expenditure even at rest. Third, maintaining a high protein intake is essential for preserving lean muscle mass during weight loss. Muscle mass is metabolically active and helps sustain a higher metabolic rate, which is beneficial for weight loss and long-term weight management.

Low-fat principles are incorporated into the diet to control calorie intake. Fats are the most calorie-dense macronutrient, with 9 calories per gram, compared to 4 calories per gram for both proteins and carbohydrates. By limiting fat intake, the diet reduces overall calorie consumption without significantly reducing the volume of food eaten. This approach also encourages the consumption of healthier fat sources, such as those found in fish, nuts, and avocados, which can support heart health without contributing excessive calories.

Incorporating these principles into daily eating habits involves choosing lean protein sources, such as chicken breast, turkey, fish, legumes, and low-fat dairy products. It also means prioritizing fruits, vegetables, and whole grains, which are nutrient-dense and can help fill up the stomach with fewer calories. Processed foods, high in sugar and unhealthy fats, are minimized as they are not only calorie-dense but also less satisfying and nutritionally poor.

Understanding and applying the low-calorie, high-protein, low-fat principles can initially seem challenging. However, with careful planning and mindful eating, it becomes manageable and can significantly contribute to achieving weight loss goals. It's not just about losing weight but also about making lifestyle changes that promote overall health and well-being.

1.1.2: Diet for Weight Loss and Health

The Dr. Nowzaradan diet, by creating a structured caloric deficit through a high-protein, low-carbohydrate, and low-fat regimen, fundamentally alters the body's metabolic processes to favor weight loss and enhance overall health. This dietary approach not only facilitates the reduction of body fat by compelling the body to utilize stored fat for energy but also supports the maintenance of lean muscle mass due to its high protein content. The preservation of muscle mass during weight loss is critical, as it prevents the metabolism from slowing down, a common issue in many weight loss programs, thereby ensuring a more sustained and effective weight management over time.

The diet's low-carbohydrate principle plays a pivotal role in managing and stabilizing blood sugar levels, which is particularly beneficial for individuals with insulin resistance or type 2 diabetes. By limiting the intake of sugars and starches, the body's insulin response is moderated, preventing the spikes and crashes in blood sugar that can lead to increased hunger and, consequently, overeating. This stabilization of blood sugar levels not only aids in the direct management of diabetes but also curtails the risk of developing the condition for those predisposed.

Furthermore, the emphasis on low-fat foods within the diet ensures that calorie intake is kept in check without necessitating the reduction of food volume. Fats, being calorically dense, contribute significantly to the total calorie count of a meal. By opting for foods low in fat, individuals can consume a larger volume of food while still adhering to the caloric limits of the diet, thereby avoiding feelings of deprivation or hunger that can often sabotage weight loss efforts. Additionally, by focusing on the consumption of healthier fats, such as those from fish, nuts, and avocados, the diet also supports cardiovascular health by improving lipid profiles and reducing the risk of heart disease.

The diet's structure and guidelines inherently encourage the consumption of nutrient-dense foods, such as vegetables, lean proteins, and whole grains, which provide essential vitamins, minerals, and fiber. This not only ensures that the body's nutritional needs are met but also promotes better digestive health and satiety between meals. The high fiber content of these foods further aids in weight loss by increasing feelings of fullness and slowing down digestion, which in turn helps to control appetite and reduce overall calorie intake.

By adhering to the principles of the Dr. Nowzaradan diet, individuals embark on a weight loss journey that is not only effective in achieving and maintaining a healthy weight but also conducive to improving overall health. The diet's balanced approach to nutrition ensures that weight loss is achieved in a healthy manner, reducing the risk of nutritional deficiencies and promoting a sustainable lifestyle change that extends beyond mere weight reduction. Through this diet, individuals gain the tools and knowledge necessary to make informed food choices that support their health and well-being in the long term.

1.1.3: Key Nutritional Guidelines

Adhering to key nutritional guidelines is essential for maximizing the benefits of the Dr. Nowzaradan diet. This diet emphasizes a balanced intake of macronutrients—proteins, carbohydrates, and fats—while ensuring a low daily caloric intake of around 1200 calories. The primary focus is on high-protein, low-carbohydrate, and low-fat foods to facilitate weight loss, improve health, and maintain muscle mass.

Proteins should be the cornerstone of each meal, as they are crucial for building and repairing tissues, and they also help in feeling full longer, which can aid in reducing overall calorie intake. Optimal sources of protein include lean meats like chicken breast, turkey, and fish, as well as plant-based options such as legumes and tofu. Incorporating a variety of these protein sources can help ensure a wide range of essential amino acids and nutrients in the diet.

Carbohydrates are necessary for energy, but it's important to choose the right kinds. Complex carbohydrates, found in whole grains, vegetables, and fruits, should be prioritized over simple carbohydrates, which are found in sugary snacks and processed foods. Complex carbohydrates provide a more sustained energy source and are packed with fiber, vitamins, and minerals. Fiber, in particular, is beneficial for digestive health and can help control blood sugar levels, contributing to longer-lasting satiety and reduced cravings.

Fats are also an essential part of the diet but should be consumed in moderation. Focus on healthy fats, such as those from avocados, nuts, seeds, and olive oil, which can support heart health without contributing to weight gain when consumed within the calorie limits of the diet. Trans fats and saturated fats, often found in processed foods, fast food, and baked goods, should be minimized as they can increase the risk of heart disease and other health issues.

In addition to macronutrients, it's vital to ensure adequate intake of vitamins and minerals, which support overall health and well-being. A diet rich in a variety of vegetables and fruits can provide most of these nutrients. However, individuals may need to consider supplementation based on their specific health needs and dietary restrictions.

Hydration is another critical aspect of the diet. Water is the best choice for staying hydrated and can aid in weight loss by helping to fill the stomach and reduce the feeling of hunger. Avoid sugary drinks and limit caffeine and alcohol, which can dehydrate the body and add unnecessary calories.

Finally, portion control is a key component of the Dr. Nowzaradan diet. Even healthy foods can contribute to weight gain if eaten in large quantities. Understanding serving sizes and using measuring tools can help manage portions effectively. Eating slowly and mindfully can also aid in recognizing fullness cues, preventing overeating.

By following these key nutritional guidelines, individuals can create a balanced, nutritious diet that supports weight loss and health improvements while adhering to the principles of the Dr. Nowzaradan diet.

1.2: GETTING STARTED

1.2.1: Setting Realistic Goals

Setting realistic goals is a fundamental step in embarking on the Dr. Nowzaradan diet. It involves understanding your current health status, acknowledging your weight loss needs, and aligning them with achievable targets within a specified timeframe. This process is not just about deciding on a number of pounds to lose; it's about creating a sustainable plan that incorporates dietary changes, physical activity, and psychological readiness for a lifestyle transformation.

Firstly, assess your current dietary habits and physical condition by keeping a food and activity journal for a week. This will provide a clear picture of where changes are needed and help set a baseline for your goals. It's crucial to be honest with yourself during this assessment to set meaningful and achievable goals.

Next, define your weight loss objectives based on the assessment. A healthy weight loss rate is typically 1-2 pounds per week. Setting a goal to lose a specific amount of weight within a realistic timeframe respects this healthy pace and contributes to long-term success. For example, aiming to lose 10 pounds in 5-10 weeks is a realistic and achievable goal for most people.

Incorporate dietary goals that focus on the principles of the Dr. Nowzaradan diet. This includes reducing your daily calorie intake to around 1200 calories, emphasizing high-protein, low-carbohydrate, and low-fat foods. Plan your meals around these guidelines, ensuring you include a variety of nutrient-dense foods to maintain balanced nutrition.

Physical activity is an essential component of weight loss and overall health. Set realistic exercise goals based on your current fitness level, gradually increasing the intensity and duration of your workouts. Starting with a goal of 30 minutes of moderate exercise, such as walking five days a week, is a practical approach for beginners.

Lastly, prepare mentally for the journey ahead. Weight loss and lifestyle changes are as much a psychological challenge as a physical one. Set goals related to improving your relationship with food, such as eating mindfully and recognizing hunger cues, to support your dietary changes. Additionally, consider setting goals for stress management and sleep improvement, as these factors significantly impact weight loss and health.

By setting realistic goals in these areas, you create a comprehensive plan that addresses all aspects of weight loss and health improvement. This holistic approach not only supports achieving your weight loss targets but also promotes a healthier, more balanced lifestyle in the long term.

1.2.2: Understanding Caloric Needs

To effectively embark on Dr. Nowzaradan's diet, understanding one's caloric needs is fundamental. This comprehension is not just about the number of calories consumed but also about the quality and nutritional value of those calories. The diet's cornerstone is a 1200-calorie-per-day regimen, designed to induce weight loss while ensuring the body receives the necessary nutrients to function optimally.

Caloric needs vary from one individual to another, influenced by factors such as age, gender, weight, height, and level of physical activity. The Basal Metabolic Rate (BMR) represents the number of calories your body needs to perform basic life-sustaining functions like breathing, circulation, cell production, and nutrient processing. Calculating your BMR is a good starting point to determine your daily caloric needs. There are several formulas to calculate BMR, including the Harris-Benedict Equation, which takes into account age, sex, weight, and height to estimate calorie requirements.

Once the BMR is established, the next step involves adjusting that number based on your activity level, known as the Total Daily Energy Expenditure (TDEE). The TDEE accounts for all physical activity, from walking to vigorous exercise. It's categorized into sedentary, lightly active, moderately active, very active, and extra active. Each category multiplies your BMR by a specific factor to estimate how many calories you burn per day, including your workouts and daily movements.

For individuals embarking on the Dr. Nowzaradan diet, the goal is to create a calorie deficit, consuming fewer calories than the body burns, leading to weight loss. However, it's crucial to ensure that the calories consumed are nutrient-dense, focusing on high-protein, low-carbohydrate, and low-fat foods. This approach not only supports weight loss but also helps in preserving muscle mass and stabilizing blood sugar levels, which is vital for overall health and well-being.

Understanding your caloric needs is a dynamic process, requiring adjustments based on weight loss progress, changes in activity levels, and other health considerations. Regular monitoring and adjustments ensure that the diet remains effective and sustainable over time, leading to successful weight management and improved health outcomes.

1.2.3: Tips for Transitioning to the Diet

Transitioning to a new diet, especially one that significantly reduces caloric intake while emphasizing high-protein, low-carbohydrate, and low-fat foods, requires a thoughtful approach to ensure success and sustainability. The following tips are designed to help individuals smoothly adapt to the dietary principles advocated by Dr. Nowzaradan, facilitating a healthier lifestyle that supports weight loss and overall well-being.

1. **Start Gradually**: Abrupt changes in diet can be overwhelming and difficult to maintain. Begin by gradually reducing portion sizes and incorporating more protein-rich foods into your meals while decreasing the intake of high-carbohydrate and high-fat foods.

2. **Plan Your Meals**: Take time each week to plan your meals. This helps in avoiding impulsive eating and ensures that you have the necessary ingredients for healthy meals. Utilize the recipes provided in this book to diversify your meal plan while adhering to the diet's guidelines.

3. **Keep a Food Diary**: Documenting what you eat can be an eye-opening experience, revealing your dietary habits and helping you stay accountable. A food diary can also assist in tracking your progress and identifying areas for improvement.

4. **Stay Hydrated**: Drinking adequate water is crucial for overall health and can aid in weight loss. Water helps in feeling full, which can reduce the likelihood of overeating. Aim for at least 8 glasses of water a day, and consider drinking a glass before meals to help control portion sizes.

5. **Seek Support**: Whether it's from family, friends, or online communities, having a support system can significantly impact your success. Sharing your goals, challenges, and achievements can provide encouragement and motivation to stay on track.

6. **Focus on Whole Foods**: Emphasize fresh vegetables, lean proteins, and whole grains in your diet. These foods are not only nutritious but also more satisfying, which can help curb cravings for processed and sugary foods.

7. **Practice Mindful Eating**: Pay attention to your hunger and fullness cues. Eat slowly, savor each bite, and learn to recognize when you're comfortably full to avoid overeating.

8. **Prepare for Challenges**: Identify potential obstacles, such as social events or dining out, and plan how to navigate them without straying from your diet. Researching restaurant menus in advance or bringing your own healthy snacks can help.

9. **Be Patient with Yourself**: Transitioning to a new diet is a process that requires time and patience. Celebrate your successes, learn from setbacks, and remember that progress is more important than perfection.

10. **Adjust as Needed**: As you progress with the diet, your nutritional needs and preferences may change. Be open to adjusting your meal plan and food choices to ensure that the diet continues to meet your needs and remains enjoyable.

By incorporating these tips into your approach to the Dr. Nowzaradan diet, you can enhance your ability to successfully transition to and maintain a healthier eating pattern that supports your weight loss and health goals.

CHAPTER 2: MEAL PLANNING AND PREPARATION

2.1: MEAL PLANNING BASICS

Meal planning is a cornerstone of maintaining a healthy diet, particularly when following Dr. Nowzaradan's 1200-calorie diet plan. It involves selecting and organizing meals in advance to meet specific nutritional goals. This process is crucial for several reasons. Firstly, it ensures that individuals consume a balanced diet that aligns with their calorie and nutritional requirements, essential for weight loss and overall health. By planning meals, individuals can avoid the pitfalls of impulsive eating decisions that often lead to unhealthy choices. Secondly, meal planning aids in grocery shopping efficiency, allowing individuals to purchase only the necessary ingredients for their planned meals, which can reduce food waste and save money. Additionally, having a meal plan helps to manage portion sizes, a key factor in controlling calorie intake. It also provides variety in the diet, preventing boredom and promoting adherence to the diet over time. Finally, meal planning can alleviate the stress associated with last-minute meal decisions, making it easier for individuals to stay committed to their health goals.

For those beginning their journey with Dr. Nowzaradan's diet, a weekly meal plan might look like this:

Breakfast
- Monday: Greek Yogurt Parfait with Berries
- Tuesday: Egg White Omelette with Spinach and Feta
- Wednesday: Cottage Cheese and Berry Bowl
- Thursday: Protein-Packed Smoothie with Almond Milk and Berries
- Friday: Turkey and Veggie Breakfast Wrap
- Saturday: Overnight Chia Pudding with Almonds
- Sunday: Smoked Salmon and Avocado Toast

Lunch
- Monday: Grilled Chicken and Veggie Wrap
- Tuesday: Tuna Salad Lettuce Wraps
- Wednesday: Turkey and Hummus Roll-Ups
- Thursday: Chicken and Quinoa Salad
- Friday: Shrimp and Avocado Salad
- Saturday: Turkey and Cucumber Roll-Ups
- Sunday: Grilled Tofu and Veggie Wrap

Dinner
- Monday: Grilled Lemon Herb Chicken
- Tuesday: Baked Cod with Asparagus
- Wednesday: Turkey and Spinach Stuffed Peppers
- Thursday: Grilled Tofu with Steamed Broccoli
- Friday: Chicken and Zucchini Noodles

- Saturday: Shrimp and Cauliflower Rice Stir-Fry
- Sunday: Turkey Meatballs with Spaghetti Squash

Dessert
- High-Protein Chocolate Lava Cake
- Greek Yogurt Cheesecake with Fresh Berries
- Protein-Packed Chocolate Chip Cookies
- Low-Fat Ricotta and Lemon Tart
- Almond Flour Chocolate Brownies
- Vanilla Protein Pudding with Cinnamon
- Berry Protein Smoothie Bowl

Nutritional values (for the previous four combined: Calories, Carbs, Fiber, Sugars, Protein, Saturated fat, Unsaturated fat):
- This will vary based on the specific recipes chosen but should align with the daily caloric goal of 1200 calories, with a focus on high protein, low carbohydrate, and low-fat foods.

Meal planning is not just about adhering to dietary restrictions; it's about creating a sustainable, healthy lifestyle that supports weight loss and health goals. By taking the time to plan meals, individuals can ensure they are nourishing their bodies with the right foods in the right amounts, setting the stage for successful weight loss and long-term health improvement.

DISCOVER THE FULL **120-DAY MEAL PLAN** STARTING ON PAGE 76.

2.2: GROCERY SHOPPING GUIDE

2.2.1: Essential Pantry Staples

Maintaining a well-stocked pantry is crucial for adhering to Dr. Nowzaradan's diet principles, ensuring that you have the necessary ingredients on hand to prepare healthy, balanced meals that align with a 1200-calorie daily intake. Focusing on high-protein, low-carbohydrate, and low-fat foods, the following list of pantry staples is designed to support your weight loss journey and overall health goals.

- **Whole Grains**: Choose whole grains such as quinoa, brown rice, and whole wheat pasta. These provide a good source of fiber and nutrients while being relatively low in calories.
- Quinoa
- Brown rice
- Whole wheat pasta
- Oats

- **Lean Proteins**: Stock up on canned or dried beans and legumes, which are excellent sources of protein and fiber. Canned tuna or salmon in water, and chicken or vegetable broth can also be used to add protein to meals without excessive calories.
- Canned beans (black beans, chickpeas, lentils)
- Canned tuna and salmon in water
- Low-sodium chicken or vegetable broth

- **Healthy Fats**: Essential for brain health and satiety, healthy fats can be found in nuts, seeds, and oils. Opt for small portions due to their high calorie density.
- Almonds, walnuts, and chia seeds
- Olive oil and avocado oil
- Natural peanut butter or almond butter

- **Low-Carb Vegetables**: Canned or frozen vegetables are convenient, nutrient-dense options that can easily be incorporated into meals. Look for options without added salt or sauces.
- Frozen spinach, broccoli, and cauliflower
- Canned tomatoes (diced or whole)
- Canned artichokes and olives

- **Condiments and Spices**: Enhance the flavor of your meals without adding unnecessary calories by using a variety of herbs, spices, and low-calorie condiments.
- Garlic powder, Italian seasoning, cumin, and chili powder
- Vinegar (balsamic, apple cider) and mustard
- Low-sodium soy sauce and salsa

- **Dairy and Dairy Alternatives**: Low-fat or fat-free options provide calcium and protein. Choose unsweetened varieties of plant-based milk for lower calorie options.
- Low-fat Greek yogurt
- Skim milk or unsweetened almond milk
- Low-fat cheese (cottage cheese, feta)

- **Eggs**: A versatile source of high-quality protein that can be used in a variety of dishes from breakfast to dinner.

- **Whole Fruit**: While fresh fruit is ideal, having canned fruit (in water or its own juice) or dried fruit (in moderation) can be a convenient alternative. Avoid options with added sugars.
- Canned peaches or pears in water
- Dried apricots or figs

By keeping these staples readily available, you can easily assemble meals that are consistent with the dietary guidelines of Dr. Nowzaradan's 1200-calorie diet plan. This approach not only aids in weight loss but also ensures that you are consuming a balanced diet rich in essential nutrients. Remember, the key to success is preparation and having the right ingredients at your fingertips.

2.2.2: Shopping Lists for the Diet

Creating a shopping list tailored to the Dr. Nowzaradan diet is essential for ensuring that you have all the necessary ingredients to prepare meals that align with the 1200-calorie daily intake goal. This diet emphasizes high-protein, low-carbohydrate, and low-fat foods to promote weight loss while ensuring nutritional needs are met. Here is a sample shopping list to help you stock your pantry, fridge, and freezer with foods that are compliant with the diet.

Proteins:
- Chicken breast (skinless)
- Turkey (ground or breast)
- Lean cuts of beef (sirloin, tenderloin)
- Fish (cod, tilapia)
- Shellfish (shrimp, scallops)
- Tofu or tempeh (for plant-based protein)
- Egg whites
- Low-fat dairy products (Greek yogurt, cottage cheese)
- Protein powder (whey or plant-based)

Vegetables:
- Leafy greens (spinach, kale, arugula)
- Broccoli
- Cauliflower
- Bell peppers
- Zucchini
- Asparagus
- Green beans
- Brussels sprouts
- Mushrooms
- Cucumbers
- Tomatoes

Fruits:
- Berries (strawberries, blueberries, raspberries)
- Apples
- Oranges
- Kiwi
- Melons
Portion Control: Due to natural sugars, fruits should be consumed in moderation

Whole Grains:
- Quinoa
- Brown rice (in moderation)
- Oats (in moderation)
- Whole grain bread (small portions).

Dairy and Dairy Alternatives:
- Low-fat Greek yogurt
- Low-fat cottage cheese
- Almond milk (unsweetened)
- Soy milk (unsweetened)

Condiments and Spices:
- Fresh herbs (parsley, cilantro, basil)
- Spices (turmeric, cumin, paprika, chili powder)
- Vinegar (apple cider, balsamic)
- Mustard
- Low-sodium soy sauce

Miscellaneous:
- Low-sodium broth (chicken, vegetable)
- Canned tomatoes (no added sugar)
- Canned beans (black beans, chickpeas - rinsed and drained)

This shopping list provides a comprehensive selection of foods that can be mixed and matched to create a variety of meals that fit within the Dr. Nowzaradan diet framework. Remember, the key to success on this diet is not just sticking to the calorie limit but also ensuring you're getting a balanced intake of nutrients. Always prioritize whole foods over processed options and pay attention to portion sizes to stay within your daily calorie goal.

2.2.3: Navigating the Grocery Store

Successfully navigating the grocery store is a crucial skill for adhering to Dr. Nowzaradan's diet plan. The layout of most stores is designed to maximize consumer spending, often leading shoppers to make impulsive, less healthy food choices. By following these strategic tips, individuals can shop more efficiently, sticking to their diet goals while avoiding common pitfalls.

1. **Stick to the Perimeter**: Most grocery stores are designed with fresh produce, dairy, and meats along the outer edges. These areas typically contain the whole, unprocessed foods that are staples of the Dr. Nowzaradan diet. Starting your shopping trip here ensures that your cart is filled with nutrient-dense, low-calorie options before you reach the more processed foods in the center aisles.

2. **Make a List and Stick to It**: Before heading to the store, plan your meals for the week and make a comprehensive shopping list. This not only saves time but also helps in resisting the temptation to buy unhealthy foods not listed. If it's not on your list, it doesn't go in the cart.

3. **Read Labels Carefully**: Understanding nutritional labels is key to making informed choices. Look for items with high protein content and low levels of sugar and saturated fat. Paying attention to serving sizes can also help you better manage your calorie intake.

4. **Shop During Off-Peak Hours**: Grocery stores are less crowded during early morning hours or late evenings on weekdays. Shopping during these times can reduce stress and give you more space to carefully choose your foods without feeling rushed.

5. **Avoid Shopping on an Empty Stomach**: Eating a small, healthy snack before grocery shopping can prevent impulsive buys driven by hunger. You're more likely to stick to your list and make healthier choices when you're not shopping on an empty stomach.

6. **Use Technology to Your Advantage**: Many grocery stores now offer apps that can help you locate items quickly, view current sales, and sometimes even see nutritional information. Using these tools can streamline your shopping process and help you make better choices.

7. **Prepare for Challenges**: The center aisles of the store can be tempting with their processed snacks and convenience foods. If you must venture into these areas for specific items like spices or whole grains, stay focused on your list and avoid lingering.

8. **Choose Frozen Wisely**: Frozen fruits and vegetables can be just as nutritious as fresh ones and last longer. However, avoid frozen meals and desserts, which can be high in calories, sugars, and unhealthy fats.

9. **Seek Out Healthier Alternatives**: Many stores now offer healthier alternatives to traditional snack foods and ingredients. Look for items like cauliflower rice, zucchini noodles, or low-carb wraps to keep your meals interesting and within your dietary guidelines.

10. **Ask for Help**: If you're having trouble finding an item, don't hesitate to ask a store employee for assistance. This can save time and prevent the frustration that might lead to making poor food choices.

By implementing these tips, grocery shopping can become a more efficient and less daunting task, supporting your journey towards weight loss and better health on Dr. Nowzaradan's diet plan.

CHAPTER 3: ENERGIZING BREAKFASTS

3.1: NUTRIENT-DENSE BREAKFAST OPTIONS

1. GREEK YOGURT WITH CUCUMBER AND HERBS

Brief Introduction

This savory Greek yogurt dish is a refreshing and nutritious way to incorporate more protein into your diet. By combining creamy low-fat Greek yogurt with fresh cucumber and herbs, this recipe offers a delicious twist to traditional yogurt parfaits, perfect for those following Dr. Now's diet principles..

Ingredients for 1 serving

- 3/4 cup non-fat Greek yogurt
- 1/4 cup cucumber, diced
- 1 tablespoon fresh dill, chopped
- 1 tablespoon fresh parsley, chopped
- 1 teaspoon lemon juice
- Salt and pepper to taste

Preparation time and Cooking time

- Preparation time: 5 minutes
- Cooking time: 0 minutes

Directions

1. In a small bowl, combine the Greek yogurt, diced cucumber, dill, parsley, and lemon juice.
2. Stir until all ingredients are well mixed.
3. Season with salt and pepper to taste.
6. Serve immediately, or refrigerate for up to 30 minutes to allow flavors to blend.

Nutritional value per serving

- Calories: 120- Carbs: 8g- Fiber: 1g- Sugars: 5g- Protein: 17g- Saturated fat: 0.5g- Unsaturated fat: 1.5g

Difficulty rating: ★★☆☆☆

2. EGG WHITE OMELETTE WITH SPINACH AND FETA

Brief Introduction

This Egg White Omelette with Spinach and Feta is a perfect start to your day, combining high-quality protein from egg whites with the nutritional powerhouse of spinach, all complemented by the tangy taste of feta cheese. This meal is designed to fit into a low-calorie, high-protein, and low-fat diet, making it an ideal choice for those following Dr. Nowzaradan's diet plan.

Ingredients for 1 serving

- 3/4 cup of egg whites
- 1 cup of fresh spinach
- 1/4 cup of crumbled feta cheese
- Salt and pepper to taste
- Non-stick cooking spray

Preparation time and Cooking time

- Preparation time: 5 minutes
- Cooking time: 5 minutes

Directions

1. Heat a non-stick skillet over medium heat and lightly coat with non-stick cooking spray.
2. While the skillet is heating, whisk the egg whites in a bowl with salt and pepper until frothy.
3. Pour the egg whites into the skillet, tilting the pan to spread them evenly.
4. As the egg whites begin to set, gently lift the edges with a spatula and tilt the pan to allow the uncooked egg whites to flow to the edges.
5. Once the egg whites are mostly set, add the fresh spinach and crumbled feta cheese to one half of the omelette.
6. Carefully fold the other half of the omelette over the filling and continue cooking for another minute, or until the cheese begins to melt and the omelette is cooked through.
7. Transfer the omelette to a plate and serve immediately.

Nutritional value per serving

- Calories: 180- Carbs: 4g- Fiber: 1g- Sugars: 2g- Protein: 26g- Saturated fat: 3g- Unsaturated fat: 0g

Difficulty rating: ★★☆☆☆

3. COTTAGE CHEESE AND BERRY BOWL

Brief Introduction

A refreshing and protein-packed start to your day, this Cottage Cheese and Berry Bowl combines the creamy texture of cottage cheese with the sweet tartness of mixed berries, creating a balanced and nutritious breakfast option.

Ingredients for 1 serving

- 1/2 cup low-fat cottage cheese
- 1/2 cup mixed berries (strawberries, blueberries, raspberries)
- 1 tablespoon sliced almonds
- 1 teaspoon stevia (optional)
- A pinch of cinnamon (optional)

Preparation time and Cooking time

- Preparation time: 5 minutes
- Cooking time: 0 minutes

Directions

1. In a serving bowl, add the low-fat cottage cheese as the base layer.
2. Top the cottage cheese with mixed berries evenly.
3. Sprinkle sliced almonds over the berries for a crunchy texture.
4. Drizzle a teaspoon of stevia over the top for added sweetness, if desired.
6. For a hint of spice, add a pinch of cinnamon over the bowl.
7. Gently mix the ingredients in the bowl before serving, if preferred, or enjoy as layered.

Nutritional value per serving

- Calories: 200- Carbs: 25g- Fiber: 2g- Sugars: 20g- Protein: 14g- Saturated fat: 1g- Unsaturated fat: 2g

Difficulty rating: ★☆☆☆☆

4. PROTEIN-PACKED SMOOTHIE WITH ALMOND MILK AND BERRIES

Brief Introduction

Start your day with a refreshing and nutritious Protein-Packed Smoothie with Almond Milk and Berries. This smoothie combines the creamy texture of almond milk with the sweet and tangy flavors of mixed berries, all while providing a high-protein kick to energize your morning without overloading on calories, fats, or sugars.

Ingredients for 1 serving

- 1 cup unsweetened almond milk
- 1/2 cup mixed berries (fresh or frozen)
- 1 scoop vanilla or plain protein powder (approximately 20-25 grams of protein)
- 1 tablespoon chia seeds

- A handful of spinach leaves (optional for extra nutrients)
- Ice cubes (optional, based on preference)

Preparation time and Cooking time

- Preparation time: 5 minutes
- Cooking time: 0 minutes

Directions

1. Place the almond milk, mixed berries, protein powder, chia seeds, and spinach leaves (if using) into a blender.
2. Add a few ice cubes if you prefer a colder smoothie.
3. Blend on high speed until the mixture is smooth and creamy, ensuring there are no lumps and the ingredients are well combined.
4. Taste the smoothie, and if needed, you can add a little more almond milk to adjust the consistency or a few drops of stevia for extra sweetness.
5. Once the smoothie reaches your desired consistency and taste, pour it into a glass and serve immediately.

Nutritional value per serving

- Calories: 230- Carbs: 18g- Fiber: 6g- Sugars: 9g- Protein: 25g- Saturated fat: 0.5g- Unsaturated fat: 2g

Difficulty rating ★★☆☆☆

5. TURKEY AND VEGGIE BREAKFAST WRAP

Brief Introduction

Start your day with a nutritious and satisfying Turkey and Veggie Breakfast Wrap. This recipe combines lean protein, fresh vegetables, and whole grains to create a balanced meal that will keep you energized throughout the morning. Perfect for those on a high-protein, low-fat diet, this wrap is both delicious and conducive to weight loss goals.

Ingredients for 1 serving:

- 1 whole wheat tortilla (low-carb option available)
- 3 oz lean turkey breast, cooked and sliced
- ¼ cup spinach, fresh
- ¼ cup bell pepper, thinly sliced
- 2 tbsp red onion, finely chopped
- 1 tbsp low-fat cream cheese
- Salt and pepper to taste
- Cooking spray (for pan)

Preparation time and Cooking time

- Preparation time: 10 minutes
- Cooking time: 5 minutes

Directions:

1. Lay the whole wheat tortilla flat on a clean surface.
2. Spread the low-fat cream cheese evenly over the tortilla.
3. Layer the sliced turkey breast on top of the cream cheese.
4. Add the fresh spinach, bell pepper, and red onion over the turkey.
5. Season with salt and pepper to taste.
6. Carefully roll the tortilla into a wrap, ensuring the fillings are securely enclosed.
7. Heat a non-stick pan over medium heat and spray lightly with cooking spray.
8. Place the wrap seam-side down in the pan and cook for 2-3 minutes until golden brown, then flip and cook the other side for an additional 2 minutes.
9. Remove from heat and let it cool for a minute before serving.

Nutritional value per serving

- Calories: 250- Carbs: 22g- Fiber: 5g- Sugars: 3g- Protein: 24g- Saturated fat: 1g- Unsaturated fat: 2g

Difficulty rating: ★★☆☆☆

6. OVERNIGHT CHIA PUDDING WITH ALMONDS

Brief Introduction

This Overnight Chia Pudding with Almonds is a perfect example of a nutrient-dense breakfast that aligns with Dr. Nowzaradan's diet principles. High in protein and fiber but low in sugars and fats, it's designed to keep you full and energized without exceeding your daily calorie limit.

Ingredients for 1 serving

- 2 tablespoons chia seeds
- 1/2 cup unsweetened almond milk
- 1/4 teaspoon vanilla extract
- 1 tablespoon sliced almonds
- 1/2 tablespoon stevia (optional, for those who prefer a bit of sweetness)
- Fresh berries for topping (optional)

Preparation time and Cooking time

- Preparation time: 5 minutes
- Cooking time: 0 minutes (overnight refrigeration)

Directions

1. In a mason jar or a small bowl, combine the chia seeds, unsweetened almond milk, and vanilla extract. Stir well to ensure the chia seeds are evenly dispersed and begin to absorb the liquid.
2. Cover the jar or bowl with a lid or plastic wrap. Refrigerate overnight, or for at least 6 hours, allowing the chia seeds to swell and the mixture to thicken into a pudding-like consistency.
3. Before serving, stir the pudding to check the consistency. If it's too thick, you can add a little more almond milk to reach your desired texture.
4. Top with sliced almonds, and if using, drizzle with stevia and add fresh berries for extra flavor and nutrients.

Nutritional value per serving

- Calories: 200- Carbs: 18g- Fiber: 9g- Sugars: 4g (without stevia)- Protein: 6g- Saturated fat: 0.5g- Unsaturated fat: 3g

Difficulty rating: ★★☆☆☆

7. SMOKED SALMON AND AVOCADO TOAST

Brief Introduction

Start your day with a balance of healthy fats, protein, and a touch of fiber with this simple yet elegant Smoked Salmon and Avocado Toast. Perfect for a quick breakfast that doesn't compromise on nutrition or taste.

Ingredients for 1 serving

- 1 slice of whole-grain bread
- 2 oz smoked salmon
- 1/4 avocado, thinly sliced
- 1 tbsp low-fat cream cheese
- 1 tsp capers
- 1/4 tsp dried dill (optional)
- Salt and pepper to taste
- A squeeze of fresh lemon juice

Preparation time and Cooking time

- Preparation time: 5 minutes
- Cooking time: 2 minutes

Directions

1. Toast the whole-grain bread to your desired level of crispiness.
2. Spread the low-fat cream cheese evenly over the toasted bread.
3. Arrange the thinly sliced avocado on top of the cream cheese.
4. Layer the smoked salmon over the avocado slices.
5. Sprinkle capers and dried dill (if using) over the smoked salmon.
6. Season with a pinch of salt and pepper to taste.
7. Finish with a squeeze of fresh lemon juice over the top for added zest.

Nutritional value per serving

- Calories: 240- Carbs: 20g- Fiber: 5g- Sugars: 3g- Protein: 15g- Saturated fat: 2g- Unsaturated fat: 5g

Difficulty rating: ★★☆☆☆

8. QUINOA BREAKFAST BOWL WITH VEGGIES

Brief Introduction

Start your day with a nutritious and energizing Quinoa Breakfast Bowl with Veggies. This recipe combines the high-protein content of quinoa with a variety of vegetables for a balanced meal that's low in fats and sugars. Perfect for those on a 1200-calorie diet plan, it's designed to keep you full and satisfied throughout the morning.

Ingredients for 1 serving

- 1/2 cup cooked quinoa
- 1/4 cup diced bell peppers
- 1/4 cup diced tomatoes
- 1/4 cup spinach leaves
- 1/4 cup chopped zucchini
- 2 tablespoons diced red onion
- 1/4 teaspoon olive oil
- Salt and pepper to taste
- 1 tablespoon fresh lemon juice
- 2 tablespoons chopped fresh herbs (such as parsley or cilantro)

Preparation time and Cooking time

- Preparation time: 10 minutes
- Cooking time: 20 minutes

Directions

1. Cook quinoa according to package instructions; set aside to cool.
2. Heat olive oil in a non-stick pan over medium heat.
3. Add red onion to the pan and sauté until translucent, about 2 minutes.

4. Add bell peppers, tomatoes, spinach, and zucchini to the pan. Season with salt and pepper. Cook until the vegetables are tender, about 5-7 minutes.
5. In a bowl, combine the cooked quinoa with the sautéed vegetables.
6. Drizzle fresh lemon juice over the quinoa and vegetable mixture.
7. Garnish with chopped fresh herbs before serving.

Nutritional value per serving

- Calories: 235- Carbs: 39g- Fiber: 6g- Sugars: 4g- Protein: 8g- Saturated fat: 0.5g- Unsaturated fat: 2g

Difficulty rating: ★★☆☆☆

9. LOW-FAT GREEK YOGURT WITH STEVIA AND WALNUTS

Ingredients for 1 serving

- 1 cup low-fat Greek yogurt
- 1 tablespoon stevia
- 2 tablespoons chopped walnuts
- 1/4 teaspoon ground cinnamon (optional)

Preparation time and Cooking time

- Preparation time: 5 minutes
- Cooking time: 0 minutes

Directions

1. Place the low-fat Greek yogurt in a serving bowl.
2. Drizzle the stevia evenly over the yogurt.
3. Sprinkle the chopped walnuts on top of the stevia.
4. If desired, add a sprinkle of ground cinnamon for extra flavor.
5. Stir the mixture gently before eating to combine the flavors.

Nutritional value per serving

- Calories: 245- Carbs: 26g- Fiber: 2g- Sugars: 23g- Protein: 20g- Saturated fat: 1g- Unsaturated fat: 5g

Difficulty rating: ★☆☆☆☆

10. SCRAMBLED TOFU WITH VEGETABLES

Brief Introduction

Start your day with a high-protein, low-fat breakfast that's both nourishing and satisfying. This scrambled tofu with vegetables recipe is a perfect example of how to incorporate a variety of nutrients into your first meal of the day, ensuring you stay full and energized without exceeding your calorie limit.

Ingredients for 1 serving

- 1/2 cup firm tofu, crumbled
- 1/4 cup red bell pepper, diced
- 1/4 cup spinach, chopped
- 1/4 cup mushrooms, sliced
- 1 tablespoon onion, finely chopped
- 1 clove garlic, minced
- 1/4 teaspoon turmeric (for color)
- Salt and pepper to taste
- 1 teaspoon olive oil

Preparation time and Cooking time

- Preparation time: 10 minutes
- Cooking time: 10 minutes

Directions

1. Heat the olive oil in a non-stick skillet over medium heat.
2. Add the onion and garlic to the skillet, sautéing until they become translucent, about 2 minutes.
3. Incorporate the mushrooms and red bell pepper into the skillet, cooking for an additional 3 minutes until they start to soften.
4. Crumble the tofu into the skillet, then sprinkle the turmeric, salt, and pepper over the mixture. Stir well to combine and evenly distribute the turmeric for color.
5. Allow the tofu to cook for about 5 minutes, stirring occasionally, until it is heated through and begins to slightly brown.
6. Add the chopped spinach and cook for another 2 minutes, or until the spinach has wilted and the ingredients are well combined.
7. Taste and adjust the seasoning if necessary before removing from heat.

Nutritional value per serving

- Calories: 200- Carbs: 10g- Fiber: 3g- Sugars: 3g- Protein: 14g- Saturated fat: 1g- Unsaturated fat: 3g

Difficulty rating: ★★☆☆☆

3.2: QUICK AND EASY BREAKFAST RECIPES

11. HIGH-PROTEIN BANANA PANCAKES

Brief Introduction

Enjoy a delicious and nutritious start to your day with these High-Protein Banana Pancakes. Perfect for those on a high-protein, low-fat diet, this recipe is designed to keep you satisfied and energized without exceeding your daily calorie goals.

Ingredients for 1 serving

- 1 medium ripe banana
- 2 large egg whites
- 1/4 cup of oat flour
- 1/2 teaspoon of baking powder
- 1/4 teaspoon of vanilla extract
- Pinch of cinnamon (optional)
- Cooking spray or a few drops of olive oil for the pan

Preparation time and Cooking time

- Preparation time: 5 minutes
- Cooking time: 10 minutes

Directions

1. Mash the ripe banana in a medium-sized bowl until smooth.
2. Add the egg whites, oat flour, baking powder, vanilla extract, and cinnamon (if using) to the mashed banana. Stir until well combined.
3. Heat a non-stick skillet over medium heat and lightly coat with cooking spray or olive oil.
4. Pour 1/4 cup of the batter onto the skillet for each pancake. Cook for about 2-3 minutes on one side, or until small bubbles form on the surface.
5. Flip the pancake carefully and cook for another 2-3 minutes on the other side until golden brown.
6. Repeat with the remaining batter, making sure to re-coat the skillet with cooking spray or oil as needed.
7. Serve the pancakes warm, with a topping of your choice that fits within the diet plan (e.g., fresh berries or a light drizzle of stevia).

Nutritional value per serving

- Calories: 240- Carbs: 42g- Fiber: 5g- Sugars: 14g- Protein: 12g- Saturated fat: 0g- Unsaturated fat: 1g

Difficulty rating: ★★☆☆☆

12. SPINACH AND MUSHROOM EGG MUFFINS

Brief Introduction

These Spinach and Mushroom Egg Muffins are a perfect grab-and-go breakfast for those busy mornings. Packed with protein and low in calories, they align with the principles of Dr. Nowzaradan's diet, offering a nutritious start to your day without compromising on flavor.

Ingredients for 1 serving

- 3 egg whites
- 1/4 cup chopped spinach
- 1/4 cup diced mushrooms
- 1 tablespoon diced red bell pepper
- Salt and pepper to taste
- Non-stick cooking spray

Preparation time and Cooking time

- Preparation time: 10 minutes
- Cooking time: 20 minutes

Directions

1. Preheat your oven to 350°F (175°C) and prepare a muffin tin by spraying it with non-stick cooking spray.
2. In a medium bowl, whisk the egg whites with salt and pepper until frothy.
3. Add the chopped spinach, diced mushrooms, and red bell pepper to the egg whites, stirring until evenly distributed.
4. Pour the egg mixture into the prepared muffin tin, filling each cup about three-quarters full.
5. Place the muffin tin in the preheated oven and bake for 20 minutes, or until the muffins are set and lightly golden on top.
6. Remove the muffin tin from the oven and allow the muffins to cool for a few minutes before removing them from the tin.
7. Serve the muffins warm, or let them cool completely and store in an airtight container for a quick breakfast throughout the week.

Nutritional value per serving

- Calories: 150- Carbs: 4g- Fiber: 1g- Sugars: 2g- Protein: 20g- Saturated fat: 0g- Unsaturated fat: 0g

Difficulty rating: ★★☆☆☆

13. TURKEY SAUSAGE AND EGG BREAKFAST BURRITO

Brief Introduction

Enjoy a delicious and nutritious start to your day with this Turkey Sausage and Egg Breakfast Burrito. Packed with protein and wrapped in a whole wheat tortilla, it's a perfect quick and easy breakfast option that aligns with a high-protein, low-fat diet.

Ingredients for 1 serving

- 1 whole wheat tortilla
- 2 egg whites
- 1 turkey sausage link, cooked and sliced
- 1/4 cup spinach, fresh
- 2 tablespoons salsa
- Salt and pepper to taste
- Non-stick cooking spray

Preparation time and Cooking time

- Preparation time: 5 minutes
- Cooking time: 10 minutes

Directions

1. Heat a non-stick skillet over medium heat and lightly coat with non-stick cooking spray.
2. In a bowl, whisk the egg whites with salt and pepper, then pour into the skillet, cooking until the eggs are set, about 3-4 minutes.
3. Warm the whole wheat tortilla in the microwave for about 10 seconds to make it more pliable.
4. Place the cooked egg whites in the center of the tortilla.
5. Top the egg whites with sliced turkey sausage and fresh spinach.
6. Add 2 tablespoons of salsa over the spinach.
7. Carefully fold the tortilla over the filling, tucking in the ends, and then roll it up tightly.
8. Place the burrito seam-side down back in the skillet and cook for 2-3 minutes on each side, or until golden brown and crispy.
9. Remove from heat and serve immediately.

Nutritional value per serving

- Calories: 250- Carbs: 18g- Fiber: 3g- Sugars: 2g- Protein: 24g- Saturated fat: 1g- Unsaturated fat: 2g

Difficulty rating: ★★☆☆☆

14. COTTAGE CHEESE AND BERRY SMOOTHIE

Brief Introduction

Kickstart your morning with a Cottage Cheese and Berry Smoothie, a perfect blend of high-protein cottage cheese and antioxidant-rich berries. This smoothie is not only quick and easy to prepare but also aligns with the nutritional guidelines of a low-calorie, high-protein, and low-fat diet, making it an ideal choice for a refreshing and energizing breakfast.

Ingredients for 1 serving

- 1/2 cup low-fat cottage cheese
- 1/2 cup mixed berries (fresh or frozen)
- 1/4 cup unsweetened almond milk
- 1 tablespoon chia seeds
- 1 teaspoon stevia (optional, for sweetness)
- Ice cubes (optional, for a colder smoothie)

Preparation time and Cooking time

- Preparation time: 5 minutes
- Cooking time: 0 minutes

Directions

1. Place the low-fat cottage cheese, mixed berries, unsweetened almond milk, and chia seeds into a blender.
2. Add stevia if a sweeter taste is desired.
3. If a colder consistency is preferred, add a few ice cubes.
4. Blend on high until the mixture is smooth and creamy, ensuring there are no lumps.
5. Taste and adjust the sweetness by adding more stevia if necessary.
6. Once the smoothie reaches your desired consistency and taste, pour it into a glass and serve immediately.

Nutritional value per serving

- Calories: 200- Carbs: 18g- Fiber: 5g- Sugars: 12g (without additional stevia)- Protein: 18g- Saturated fat: 0.5g- Unsaturated fat: 1g

Difficulty rating: ★☆☆☆☆

15. ALMOND BUTTER AND BANANA RICE CAKES

Brief Introduction

Enjoy a simple, nutritious, and quick breakfast with Almond Butter and Banana Rice Cakes. This recipe combines the creamy texture of almond butter with the natural sweetness of banana, topped on a crispy rice cake for a satisfying crunch. It's an excellent source of protein and healthy fats, making it a perfect fit for a low-calorie, high-protein diet.

Ingredients for 1 serving

- 2 plain rice cakes
- 2 tablespoons almond butter
- 1 medium banana, sliced
- 1/4 teaspoon cinnamon (optional)
- 1 teaspoon stevia (optional)

Preparation time and Cooking time

- Preparation time: 5 minutes
- Cooking time: 0 minutes

Directions

1. Spread 1 tablespoon of almond butter evenly over each rice cake.
2. Arrange the banana slices on top of the almond butter on each rice cake.
3. If desired, sprinkle cinnamon over the banana slices for added flavor.
4. Drizzle a small amount of stevia over each rice cake for a touch of sweetness, if using.
5. Serve immediately for the best texture and flavor.

Nutritional value per serving

- Calories: 245- Carbs: 38g- Fiber: 5g- Sugars: 17g- Protein: 6g- Saturated fat: 1g
- Unsaturated fat: 4g

Difficulty rating: ★☆☆☆☆

16. LOW-FAT RICOTTA AND BERRY TOAST

Brief Introduction

Elevate your morning routine with this Low-Fat Ricotta and Berry Toast, a delightful combination of creamy ricotta, juicy berries, and whole-grain toast. This recipe is designed to fit into a high-protein, low-fat diet, making it an ideal choice for a quick and nutritious breakfast.

Ingredients for 1 serving

- 1 slice of whole-grain bread
- 1/4 cup low-fat ricotta cheese

- 1/2 cup mixed berries (such as strawberries, blueberries, and raspberries)
- 1 teaspoon stevia (optional)
- A pinch of cinnamon (optional)

Preparation time and Cooking time

- Preparation time: 5 minutes
- Cooking time: 2 minutes

Directions

1. Toast the slice of whole-grain bread to your desired level of crispiness.
2. Spread the low-fat ricotta cheese evenly over the toasted bread.
3. Arrange the mixed berries on top of the ricotta.
4. If desired, drizzle stevia over the berries for added sweetness.
5. Sprinkle a pinch of cinnamon over the toast for extra flavor.
6. Serve immediately while the toast is still warm.

Nutritional value per serving

- Calories: 200- Carbs: 28g- Fiber: 5g- Sugars: 12g- Protein: 12g- Saturated fat: 1g- Unsaturated fat: 1g

Difficulty rating: ★☆☆☆☆

17. PROTEIN-PACKED VEGGIE SCRAMBLE

Brief Introduction

Energize your morning with this Protein-Packed Veggie Scramble, a perfect blend of high-quality protein and fiber-rich vegetables to kickstart your day without breaking your calorie bank. This recipe aligns with the principles of high protein, low fat, and low sugar, making it an ideal choice for a nutritious breakfast.

Ingredients for 1 serving

- 1/2 cup egg whites

- 1/4 cup diced bell peppers (mix of red, yellow, and green for color and flavor)
- 1/4 cup chopped spinach
- 1/4 cup sliced mushrooms
- 2 tablespoons diced onions
- 1 clove garlic, minced
- Salt and pepper to taste
- 1 teaspoon olive oil

Preparation time and Cooking time

- Preparation time: 5 minutes
- Cooking time: 10 minutes

Directions

1. Heat the olive oil in a non-stick skillet over medium heat.
2. Add the onions and garlic to the skillet, sautéing until the onions become translucent, about 2 minutes.
3. Incorporate the bell peppers and mushrooms into the skillet, cooking for an additional 3 minutes until they start to soften.
4. Stir in the chopped spinach and cook until it wilts, approximately 2 minutes.
5. Pour the egg whites over the sautéed vegetables, seasoning with salt and pepper.
6. Allow the egg whites to set on the bottom, then gently stir to combine with the vegetables, cooking until the egg whites are fully cooked, about 3 minutes.
7. Serve immediately while hot.

Nutritional value per serving

- Calories: 150- Carbs: 8g- Fiber: 2g- Sugars: 4g- Protein: 18g- Saturated fat: 0.5g- Unsaturated fat: 2g

Difficulty rating: ★★☆☆☆

18. CHICKEN AND AVOCADO BREAKFAST SALAD

Brief Introduction

This Chicken and Avocado Breakfast Salad is a refreshing and protein-rich way to start your day. Combining lean chicken breast with creamy avocado and a variety of greens, this salad is not only satisfying but also aligns with the principles of a high-protein, low-fat diet. Perfect for those looking to maintain a balanced diet without compromising on flavor.

Ingredients for 1 serving

- 3 oz grilled chicken breast, diced
- 1/2 ripe avocado, cubed
- 1 cup mixed salad greens (such as spinach, arugula, and romaine)
- 1/4 cup cherry tomatoes, halved
- 1 tablespoon red onion, finely chopped
- 1 tablespoon lemon juice
- Salt and pepper to taste
- 1 teaspoon olive oil

Preparation time and Cooking time

- Preparation time: 10 minutes
- Cooking time: 0 minutes

Directions

1. In a large mixing bowl, combine the mixed salad greens, cherry tomatoes, and red onion.
2. Add the cubed avocado and diced grilled chicken breast to the bowl.
3. In a small bowl, whisk together the lemon juice, olive oil, salt, and pepper to create the dressing.
4. Drizzle the dressing over the salad and gently toss to ensure all ingredients are evenly coated.
5. Serve the salad immediately to enjoy the freshness of the ingredients.

Nutritional value per serving

- Calories: 250- Carbs: 9g- Fiber: 5g- Sugars: 2g- Protein: 25g- Saturated fat: 2g
- Unsaturated fat: 5g

Difficulty rating: ★★☆☆☆

19. LOW-FAT GREEK YOGURT WITH FRESH FRUIT

Brief Introduction

Enjoy a refreshing and protein-rich start to your day with this Low-Fat Greek Yogurt with Fresh Fruit recipe. Combining the creamy texture of Greek yogurt with the natural sweetness of fresh fruit, this breakfast option is not only delicious but also aligns with the principles of a high-protein, low-fat diet. It's quick to prepare, making it an ideal choice for a nutritious morning meal.

Ingredients for 1 serving

- 1 cup low-fat Greek yogurt
- 1/2 cup mixed fresh berries (such as strawberries, blueberries, and raspberries)
- 1 tablespoon sliced almonds
- 1 teaspoon stevia (optional)

Preparation time and Cooking time

- Preparation time: 5 minutes
- Cooking time: 0 minutes

Directions

1. Spoon the low-fat Greek yogurt into a serving bowl.
2. Top the yogurt with the mixed fresh berries.
3. Sprinkle the sliced almonds over the berries.
4. If desired, drizzle stevia over the top for added sweetness.
5. Gently mix the ingredients together before enjoying, or layer them beautifully for a visually appealing breakfast.

Nutritional value per serving

- Calories: 230- Carbs: 25g- Fiber: 4g- Sugars: 18g- Protein: 20g- Saturated fat: 1g- Unsaturated fat: 2g

Difficulty rating: ★☆☆☆☆

20. EGG WHITE AND VEGGIE BREAKFAST SANDWICH

Brief Introduction

Elevate your morning routine with this Egg White and Veggie Breakfast Sandwich. Packed with protein and loaded with fresh vegetables, it's a nutritious and satisfying way to start your day within the parameters of a low-calorie, high-protein, and low-fat diet.

Ingredients for 1 serving

- 3/4 cup of egg whites
- 1 whole grain English muffin
- 1/4 cup of spinach, fresh
- 2 slices of tomato
- 1 slice of low-fat cheese
- Salt and pepper to taste
- Non-stick cooking spray

Preparation time and Cooking time

- Preparation time: 5 minutes
- Cooking time: 10 minutes

Directions

1. Preheat a non-stick skillet over medium heat and lightly coat with non-stick cooking spray.
2. Pour the egg whites into the skillet, seasoning with salt and pepper. Cook until the egg whites are fully set, flipping once to ensure even cooking.
3. While the egg whites are cooking, split the English muffin and toast it to your preference.
4. Once the egg whites are done, place them on the bottom half of the toasted English muffin.
5. Layer the fresh spinach and tomato slices on top of the egg whites.
6. Add a slice of low-fat cheese atop the vegetables.
7. Cap with the other half of the English muffin, pressing down gently to secure the layers.
8. Serve immediately while warm.

Nutritional value per serving

- Calories: 250- Carbs: 28g- Fiber: 6g- Sugars: 4g- Protein: 26g- Saturated fat: 1g
- Unsaturated fat: 2g

Difficulty rating: ★★☆☆☆

CHAPTER 4: SATISFYING LUNCHES

4.1: PORTABLE OPTIONS FOR BUSY DAYS

21. GRILLED CHICKEN AND VEGGIE WRAP

Brief Introduction

This Grilled Chicken and Veggie Wrap is a flavorful, nutritious option for a quick lunch. Packed with lean protein and fresh vegetables, it's perfectly aligned with a high-protein, low-fat diet, making it an ideal choice for those busy days when time is of the essence but health is still a priority.

Ingredients for 1 serving

- 3 oz grilled chicken breast, thinly sliced
- 1 whole wheat tortilla (8-inch diameter)
- ¼ cup mixed bell peppers, thinly sliced
- ¼ cup spinach leaves, fresh
- 2 tbsp red onion, thinly sliced
- 1 tbsp low-fat Greek yogurt
- 1 tsp Dijon mustard
- Salt and pepper to taste
- Non-stick cooking spray

Preparation time and Cooking time

- Preparation time: 10 minutes
- Cooking time: 5 minutes

Directions

1. Preheat a grill pan over medium heat and lightly coat with non-stick cooking spray.
2. Grill the sliced bell peppers and red onion until they are slightly charred and tender, about 3-4 minutes, then set aside.
3. In a small bowl, mix the low-fat Greek yogurt and Dijon mustard together. Season with salt and pepper to taste.
4. Lay the whole wheat tortilla flat on a plate and spread the Greek yogurt and mustard mixture evenly over the surface.
5. Arrange the grilled chicken slices down the center of the tortilla.
6. Top the chicken with the grilled bell peppers, red onion, and fresh spinach leaves.
7. Carefully roll the tortilla, folding in the sides first to enclose the filling, then rolling from the bottom up tightly.
8. Place the wrap back on the grill pan, seam side down, and grill for about 1-2 minutes on each side or until the wrap is heated through and has grill marks.
9. Remove from heat and slice the wrap in half diagonally before serving.

Nutritional value per serving

- Calories: 300- Carbs: 28g- Fiber: 5g- Sugars: 3g- Protein: 26g- Saturated fat: 1g
- Unsaturated fat: 2g

Difficulty rating: ★★☆☆☆

22. TUNA SALAD LETTUCE WRAPS

Brief Introduction

These Tuna Salad Lettuce Wraps are a light, refreshing, and protein-packed lunch option, perfect for those busy days when you need a quick yet nutritious meal. High in protein and low in both fats and sugars, they align perfectly with the dietary guidelines of a 1200-

calorie diet plan, offering a satisfying meal without the guilt.

Ingredients for 1 serving

- 1 can (5 oz) tuna in water, drained
- 1/4 cup non-fat Greek yogurt
- 1 tablespoon Dijon mustard
- 1/4 cup diced celery
- 1/4 cup diced red onion
- Salt and pepper to taste
- 4 large lettuce leaves (such as romaine or butter lettuce)
- 2 tablespoons chopped fresh herbs (such as parsley or chives, optional)

Preparation time and Cooking time

- Preparation time: 10 minutes
- Cooking time: 0 minutes

Directions

1. In a medium bowl, mix together the drained tuna, non-fat Greek yogurt, and Dijon mustard until well combined.
2. Stir in the diced celery and red onion. Season the mixture with salt and pepper according to your taste preferences.
3. Carefully wash and dry the lettuce leaves, ensuring they are clean and intact for wrapping.
4. Divide the tuna salad evenly among the lettuce leaves, placing a scoop in the center of each leaf.
5. If using, sprinkle the chopped fresh herbs over the tuna salad for added flavor.
6. To serve, fold the lettuce leaves around the tuna salad, creating a wrap. Enjoy immediately for the best texture and freshness.

Nutritional value per serving

- Calories: 200- Carbs: 6g- Fiber: 2g- Sugars: 3g- Protein: 33g- Saturated fat: 0g
- Unsaturated fat: 1g

Difficulty rating: ★☆☆☆☆

23. TURKEY AND HUMMUS ROLL-UPS

Brief Introduction

These Turkey and Hummus Roll-Ups are a perfect high-protein, low-fat, and low-sugar lunch option that is both delicious and satisfying. Ideal for busy days, they are quick to prepare, easy to transport, and can be enjoyed anywhere, making them a fantastic choice for a nutritious meal on the go.

Ingredients for 1 serving

- 3 slices of low-fat turkey breast
- 2 tablespoons hummus
- 1 whole wheat tortilla (8-inch diameter)
- 1/4 cup spinach leaves, fresh
- 1/4 cup shredded carrots
- 1/4 cup cucumber, thinly sliced
- Salt and pepper to taste

Preparation time and Cooking time

- Preparation time: 10 minutes
- Cooking time: 0 minutes

Directions

1. Lay the whole wheat tortilla flat on a clean surface.
2. Spread the hummus evenly over the surface of the tortilla.
3. Arrange the turkey slices on top of the hummus, covering the tortilla evenly.
4. Layer the spinach leaves, shredded carrots, and cucumber slices over the turkey.
5. Season with a pinch of salt and pepper to taste.
6. Carefully roll the tortilla tightly, ensuring the fillings are securely wrapped inside.
7. Once rolled, cut the roll-up into halves or bite-sized pieces, depending on preference.
8. Serve immediately, or wrap in foil to maintain freshness if taking on the go.

Nutritional value per serving

- Calories: 320- Carbs: 35g- Fiber: 5g- Sugars: 3g- Protein: 24g- Saturated fat: 1g
- Unsaturated fat: 2g

Difficulty rating: ★★☆☆☆

24. CHICKEN AND QUINOA SALAD

Brief Introduction

This Chicken and Quinoa Salad is a vibrant, nutritious dish perfect for a satisfying lunch. High in protein and packed with a variety of vegetables, it's designed to keep you energized throughout the day while adhering to a low-calorie, high-protein, and low-fat diet.

Ingredients for 1 serving

- 1/2 cup cooked quinoa
- 3 oz grilled chicken breast, chopped
- 1/4 cup cherry tomatoes, halved
- 1/4 cup cucumber, diced
- 1/4 cup red bell pepper, diced
- 2 tablespoons red onion, finely chopped
- 1 tablespoon fresh parsley, chopped
- 1 tablespoon lemon juice
- 1 teaspoon olive oil
- Salt and pepper to taste

Preparation time and Cooking time

- Preparation time: 15 minutes
- Cooking time: 0 minutes (assuming quinoa and chicken are pre-cooked)

Directions

1. In a large mixing bowl, combine the cooked quinoa, chopped grilled chicken, halved cherry tomatoes, diced cucumber, diced red bell pepper, and finely chopped red onion.
2. Add the chopped fresh parsley to the bowl for a fresh flavor.
3. In a small bowl, whisk together the lemon juice, olive oil, salt, and pepper to create a light dressing.
4. Pour the dressing over the salad ingredients in the large bowl. Toss everything together until the salad is evenly coated with the dressing.
5. Taste and adjust the seasoning if necessary, adding more salt, pepper, or lemon juice as desired.
6. Serve the salad immediately, or refrigerate it for an hour to allow the flavors to meld together for an even more delicious experience.

Nutritional value per serving

- Calories: 330- Carbs: 27g- Fiber: 5g- Sugars: 4g- Protein: 28g- Saturated fat: 1g
- Unsaturated fat: 3g

Difficulty rating: ★★☆☆☆

25. SHRIMP AND AVOCADO SALAD

Brief Introduction

This Shrimp and Avocado Salad is a refreshing and protein-rich meal, perfect for a satisfying lunch that's easy to prepare on busy days. Combining succulent shrimp with creamy avocado and a zesty lime dressing, it's a delicious way to stay on track with your low-calorie, high-protein diet goals.

Ingredients for 1 serving

- 4 oz cooked shrimp, peeled and deveined
- 1/2 ripe avocado, cubed
- 1 cup mixed greens (such as arugula, spinach, and romaine)
- 1/4 cup cherry tomatoes, halved
- 1 tablespoon red onion, finely chopped
- 2 tablespoons cilantro, chopped
- Juice of 1 lime
- 1 teaspoon olive oil
- Salt and pepper to taste

Preparation time and Cooking time

- Preparation time: 10 minutes
- Cooking time: 0 minutes

Directions

1. In a large mixing bowl, combine the mixed greens, cherry tomatoes, and red onion.
2. Add the cubed avocado and cooked shrimp to the bowl.
3. In a small bowl, whisk together the lime juice, olive oil, salt, and pepper to create the dressing.
4. Drizzle the dressing over the salad ingredients in the large bowl.
5. Gently toss the salad to ensure all ingredients are evenly coated with the dressing.
6. Sprinkle chopped cilantro over the top of the salad for added flavor.
7. Serve the salad immediately, or cover and refrigerate for up to 2 hours before serving to allow flavors to meld.

Nutritional value per serving

- Calories: 320- Carbs: 14g- Fiber: 7g- Sugars: 2g- Protein: 25g- Saturated fat: 2g
- Unsaturated fat: 10g

Difficulty rating: ★★☆☆☆

26. TURKEY AND CUCUMBER ROLL-UPS

Brief Introduction

These Turkey and Cucumber Roll-Ups are a refreshing, protein-packed lunch option that's perfect for those busy days when you need a quick, nutritious meal. With lean turkey breast and crisp cucumber, these roll-ups are low in calories but high in flavor, aligning with the principles of a high-protein, low-fat diet.

Ingredients for 1 serving

- 3 oz lean turkey breast slices
- 1/2 medium cucumber, thinly sliced lengthwise
- 1 tablespoon hummus
- 1/4 cup spinach leaves
- Salt and pepper to taste

Preparation time and Cooking time

- Preparation time: 10 minutes
- Cooking time: 0 minutes

Directions

1. Lay out the turkey breast slices flat on a clean surface.
2. Spread a thin layer of hummus over each turkey slice.
3. Arrange a few spinach leaves on one end of each turkey slice.
4. Place a few cucumber slices on top of the spinach.
5. Season with salt and pepper.
6. Carefully roll up the turkey slices tightly, starting from the end with the spinach and cucumber.
7. Secure each roll-up with a toothpick if necessary.
8. Serve immediately or store in the refrigerator until ready to eat.

Nutritional value per serving

- Calories: 150- Carbs: 4g- Fiber: 1g- Sugars: 2g- Protein: 25g- Saturated fat: 0.5g
- Unsaturated fat: 1g

Difficulty rating: ★☆☆☆☆

27. GRILLED TOFU AND VEGGIE WRAP

Brief Introduction

This Grilled Tofu and Veggie Wrap is a flavorful, nutritious option for a quick lunch. High in protein and packed with fresh vegetables, it's perfectly aligned with a low-calorie, high-protein, and low-fat diet, making it an ideal choice for those busy days when you need a portable yet satisfying meal.

Ingredients for 1 serving

- 1/2 cup firm tofu, pressed and sliced into strips
- 1 whole wheat tortilla
- 1/4 cup bell peppers, thinly sliced
- 1/4 cup zucchini, thinly sliced

- 1/4 cup red onion, thinly sliced
- 1 tablespoon low-sodium soy sauce
- 1 teaspoon olive oil
- 1/4 teaspoon garlic powder
- 1/4 teaspoon ground black pepper
- 1/2 cup spinach leaves

Preparation time and Cooking time

- Preparation time: 15 minutes
- Cooking time: 10 minutes

Directions

1. Marinate the tofu strips in soy sauce, garlic powder, and black pepper for at least 10 minutes.
2. Heat olive oil in a grill pan over medium heat.
3. Add the marinated tofu strips to the grill pan and cook for about 2-3 minutes on each side, or until they have grill marks and are heated through. Remove from the pan and set aside.
4. In the same pan, add bell peppers, zucchini, and red onion, grilling them for about 2-3 minutes or until they are slightly softened but still crisp.
5. Warm the whole wheat tortilla in a microwave for about 10 seconds to make it more pliable.
6. Lay the tortilla flat and arrange the grilled tofu strips down the center.
7. Top the tofu with the grilled vegetables and fresh spinach leaves.
8. Carefully roll the tortilla around the fillings, folding in the sides to secure the wrap.
9. Cut the wrap in half, if desired, and serve immediately or wrap in foil to take on the go.

Nutritional value per serving

- Calories: 330- Carbs: 35g- Fiber: 6g- Sugars: 5g- Protein: 18g- Saturated fat: 1g
- Unsaturated fat: 3g

Difficulty rating: ★★☆☆☆

28. CHICKEN AND BLACK BEAN SALAD

Brief Introduction

This Chicken and Black Bean Salad is a vibrant, protein-packed dish that's perfect for a quick lunch on a busy day. Combining lean chicken breast with fiber-rich black beans and a variety of fresh vegetables, it's a nutritious meal that aligns with the high-protein, low-fat principles of the diet.

Ingredients for 1 serving

- 3 oz cooked chicken breast, diced
- 1/2 cup black beans, rinsed and drained
- 1 cup mixed greens (such as lettuce, spinach, and arugula)
- 1/4 cup cherry tomatoes, halved
- 1/4 cup cucumber, diced
- 1/4 avocado, diced
- 2 tablespoons red onion, finely chopped
- 1 tablespoon cilantro, chopped
- 1 tablespoon lime juice
- Salt and pepper to taste
- 1 teaspoon olive oil

Preparation time and Cooking time

- Preparation time: 15 minutes
- Cooking time: 0 minutes

Directions

1. In a large mixing bowl, combine the mixed greens, cherry tomatoes, cucumber, avocado, and red onion.
2. Add the diced chicken breast and black beans to the bowl.
3. In a small bowl, whisk together the lime juice, olive oil, salt, and pepper to create the dressing.
4. Drizzle the dressing over the salad and toss gently to ensure all ingredients are evenly coated.
5. Garnish with chopped cilantro before serving.
6. Adjust salt and pepper to taste, if necessary.

Nutritional value per serving

- Calories: 345- Carbs: 32g- Fiber: 10g-
Sugars: 3g- Protein: 28g- Saturated fat: 2g
- Unsaturated fat: 5g

Difficulty rating: ★★☆☆☆

29. TURKEY AND SPINACH PINWHEELS

Brief Introduction

These Turkey and Spinach Pinwheels are a
delightful and nutritious option for a quick
lunch. Packed with lean protein from turkey
and vitamins from spinach, wrapped in a
whole wheat tortilla, they are perfect for those
on the go. Following the principles of high
protein and low fat, these pinwheels are both
satisfying and aligned with a 1200-calorie diet
plan.

Ingredients for 1 serving

- 1 whole wheat tortilla (8-inch)
- 3 oz thinly sliced turkey breast
- 1/2 cup fresh spinach leaves
- 2 tablespoons low-fat cream cheese, softened
- 1 tablespoon red bell pepper, finely diced
- Salt and pepper to taste

Preparation time and Cooking time

- Preparation time: 10 minutes
- Cooking time: 0 minutes

Directions

1. Lay the whole wheat tortilla flat on a clean
surface.
2. Spread the low-fat cream cheese evenly over
the entire surface of the tortilla.
3. Arrange the thinly sliced turkey breast over
the cream cheese, covering most of the tortilla.
4. Distribute the fresh spinach leaves and
diced red bell pepper evenly on top of the
turkey slices.
5. Season with a pinch of salt and pepper to
taste.
6. Carefully roll the tortilla tightly, starting
from one edge and working your way to the
other side to ensure the fillings are securely
wrapped.
7. Once rolled, use a sharp knife to slice the
tortilla roll into 1-inch thick pinwheels.
8. Serve immediately or store in an airtight
container for a portable lunch option.

Nutritional value per serving

- Calories: 320- Carbs: 35g- Fiber: 5g- Sugars:
3g- Protein: 25g- Saturated fat: 2g
- Unsaturated fat: 2g

Difficulty rating: ★★☆☆☆

30. GRILLED SHRIMP AND VEGGIE SKEWERS

Brief Introduction

Enjoy a light and flavorful meal with these
Grilled Shrimp and Veggie Skewers. Perfect
for a high-protein, low-fat diet, these skewers
are packed with nutrients and can be prepared
quickly, making them an ideal choice for a
satisfying lunch on busy days.

Ingredients for 1 serving

- 6 large shrimp, peeled and deveined
- 1/2 bell pepper, cut into 1-inch pieces
- 1/2 zucchini, cut into 1/2-inch thick rounds
- 1/2 red onion, cut into wedges
- 1 tablespoon olive oil
- 1 garlic clove, minced
- Salt and pepper to taste
- 1/2 teaspoon smoked paprika
- 2 wooden or metal skewers

Preparation time and Cooking time

- Preparation time: 15 minutes
- Cooking time: 10 minutes

Directions

1. If using wooden skewers, soak them in water
for at least 30 minutes to prevent burning.
2. Preheat the grill to medium-high heat.

3. In a large bowl, combine the olive oil, minced garlic, salt, pepper, and smoked paprika.

4. Add the shrimp, bell pepper, zucchini, and red onion to the bowl. Toss to coat the ingredients evenly with the seasoning.

5. Thread the shrimp and vegetables alternately onto the skewers.

6. Place the skewers on the grill. Cook for 2-3 minutes on each side or until the shrimp turn pink and the vegetables are slightly charred.

7. Remove the skewers from the grill and allow them to rest for a couple of minutes before serving.

Nutritional value per serving

- Calories: 300- Carbs: 12g- Fiber: 3g- Sugars: 5g- Protein: 25g- Saturated fat: 1.5g
- Unsaturated fat: 5g

Difficulty rating: ★★☆☆☆

4.2: SIMPLE AND SATISFYING LUNCH RECIPES

31. GRILLED CHICKEN CAESAR SALAD

Brief Introduction

This Grilled Chicken Caesar Salad combines lean protein, crisp romaine lettuce, and a light Caesar dressing for a refreshing and satisfying lunch. Perfect for those following a high-protein, low-fat diet, this salad is both delicious and nutritious.

Ingredients for 1 serving

- 3 oz grilled chicken breast, sliced
- 2 cups romaine lettuce, chopped
- 2 tablespoons low-fat Caesar dressing
- 1 tablespoon grated Parmesan cheese
- 1/4 cup whole wheat croutons
- Lemon wedge for garnish
- Black pepper to taste

Preparation time and Cooking time

- Preparation time: 10 minutes
- Cooking time: 10 minutes (for the chicken, if not pre-cooked)

Directions

1. If the chicken breast is not yet cooked, preheat a grill or grill pan over medium heat. Season the chicken breast with black pepper and place it on the grill. Cook for 5 minutes on each side or until the internal temperature reaches 165°F. Allow it to rest for a few minutes before slicing.
2. In a large bowl, toss the chopped romaine lettuce with the low-fat Caesar dressing until the lettuce is evenly coated.
3. Add the sliced grilled chicken on top of the dressed lettuce.
4. Sprinkle the grated Parmesan cheese over the salad.
5. Add the whole wheat croutons for a crunchy texture.
6. Garnish with a lemon wedge and additional black pepper to taste.
7. Serve immediately for the freshest flavor.

Nutritional value per serving

- Calories: 300- Carbs: 18g- Fiber: 3g- Sugars: 3g- Protein: 28g- Saturated fat: 3g
- Unsaturated fat: 4g

Difficulty rating: ★★☆☆☆

32. SPICY TUNA AND AVOCADO WRAP

Brief Introduction

Elevate your lunchtime with this Spicy Tuna and Avocado Wrap, a perfect blend of protein-rich tuna, creamy avocado, and a kick of spice. This wrap is not only flavorful but also aligns with a high-protein, low-fat diet, making it an ideal choice for a nutritious and satisfying meal.

Ingredients for 1 serving

- 1 whole wheat tortilla (8-inch diameter)
- 3 oz canned tuna in water, drained
- 1/4 ripe avocado, mashed
- 1 tbsp low-fat Greek yogurt
- 1/2 tbsp Sriracha sauce (adjust to taste)
- 1/4 cup mixed greens (spinach, arugula, etc.)
- 2 tbsp diced red bell pepper
- Salt and pepper to taste

Preparation time and Cooking time

- Preparation time: 10 minutes
- Cooking time: 0 minutes

Directions

1. Lay the whole wheat tortilla flat on a clean surface.
2. In a small bowl, mix the drained tuna, mashed avocado, low-fat Greek yogurt, and Sriracha sauce. Season with salt and pepper to taste.
3. Spread the tuna mixture evenly over the center of the tortilla, leaving a small border around the edges.
4. Sprinkle the mixed greens and diced red bell pepper on top of the tuna mixture.
5. Carefully roll the tortilla, folding in the sides first to enclose the filling, then rolling from the bottom up tightly.
6. Cut the wrap in half diagonally and serve immediately or wrap in foil to take on the go.

Nutritional value per serving

- Calories: 330- Carbs: 27g- Fiber: 5g- Sugars: 3g- Protein: 25g- Saturated fat: 1g
- Unsaturated fat: 3g

Difficulty rating: ★★☆☆☆

33. LEMON HERB QUINOA SALAD

Brief Introduction

A vibrant and refreshing dish that's as nutritious as it is flavorful. Packed with protein-rich quinoa and infused with the zesty freshness of lemon and herbs, this salad is the perfect balance of light yet satisfying. Whether you're looking for a wholesome lunch or a healthy side, this recipe is a delicious way to stay on track with your weight loss goals while enjoying a burst of flavor.

Ingredients for 1 serving

- 1/2 cup cooked quinoa
- 1/4 cup diced cucumber
- 1/4 cup cherry tomatoes, halved
- 1/4 cup diced red bell pepper
- 2 tablespoons diced red onion
- 2 tablespoons chopped fresh parsley
- 1 tablespoon extra virgin olive oil
- Juice of 1/2 lemon
- 1/4 teaspoon dried oregano
- Salt and pepper to taste

Preparation time and Cooking time

- Preparation time: 10 minutes
- Cooking time: 0 minutes (assuming quinoa is pre-cooked)

Directions

1. In a large mixing bowl, combine the cooked quinoa, diced cucumber, halved cherry tomatoes, diced red bell pepper, and diced red onion.
2. Add the chopped fresh parsley to the bowl for a fresh flavor.
3. In a small bowl, whisk together the extra virgin olive oil, lemon juice, dried oregano, salt, and pepper to create the dressing.
4. Pour the dressing over the quinoa and vegetable mixture. Toss everything together until the salad is evenly coated with the dressing.
5. Taste and adjust the seasoning if necessary, adding more salt, pepper, or lemon juice as desired.
6. Serve the salad immediately, or let it chill in the refrigerator for about 30 minutes to allow the flavors to meld together.

Nutritional value per serving

- Calories: 330- Carbs: 40g- Fiber: 5g- Sugars: 4g- Protein: 8g- Saturated fat: 1g
- Unsaturated fat: 5g

Difficulty rating: ★★☆☆☆

34. TURKEY AND APPLE SANDWICH

Brief Introduction

A deliciously simple yet flavorful combination of lean turkey, crisp apple slices, and whole-grain bread. This high-protein, low-fat sandwich is the perfect balance of savory and sweet, making it a great choice for a healthy lunch or snack.

Ingredients for 1 serving
- 2 slices of whole-grain bread
- 3 oz thinly sliced turkey breast
- 1/2 apple, thinly sliced
- 1 tablespoon mustard
- 1/4 cup spinach leaves
- Salt and pepper to taste

Preparation time and Cooking time
- Preparation time: 5 minutes
- Cooking time: 0 minutes

Directions
1. Lay out the two slices of whole-grain bread on a clean surface.
2. Spread the mustard evenly on one slice of bread.
3. Arrange the thinly sliced turkey breast over the mustard.
4. Place the thinly sliced apple pieces on top of the turkey.
5. Add the spinach leaves over the apple slices. Season with a pinch of salt and pepper.
6. Cover with the second slice of bread.
7. Cut the sandwich in half, if desired, and serve immediately.

Nutritional value per serving
- Calories: 330- Carbs: 40g- Fiber: 6g- Sugars: 12g- Protein: 25g- Saturated fat: 1g
- Unsaturated fat: 2g

Difficulty rating: ★☆☆☆☆

35. CHICKPEA AND VEGGIE SALAD

Brief Introduction

A hearty, nutrient-packed dish featuring protein-rich chickpeas combined with a colorful mix of fresh vegetables. Bursting with flavors and textures, this salad offers a satisfying, low-calorie meal that is both filling and nutritious.

Ingredients for 1 serving
- 1/2 cup chickpeas, rinsed and drained
- 1 cup mixed greens (spinach, arugula, and romaine)
- 1/4 cup cherry tomatoes, halved
- 1/4 cucumber, diced
- 1/4 red bell pepper, diced
- 2 tablespoons red onion, finely chopped
- 1 tablespoon fresh parsley, chopped
- 1 tablespoon lemon juice
- 1 teaspoon olive oil
- Salt and pepper to taste

Preparation time and Cooking time
- Preparation time: 10 minutes
- Cooking time: 0 minutes

Directions
1. In a large mixing bowl, combine the chickpeas, mixed greens, cherry tomatoes, cucumber, red bell pepper, and red onion.
2. Add the chopped parsley to the bowl for a fresh flavor.
3. In a small bowl, whisk together the lemon juice, olive oil, salt, and pepper to create a light dressing.
4. Pour the dressing over the salad ingredients in the large bowl. Toss everything together until the salad is evenly coated with the dressing.
5. Taste and adjust the seasoning if necessary, adding more salt, pepper, or lemon juice as desired.
6. Serve the salad immediately, or let it chill in the refrigerator for about 30 minutes to enhance the flavors.

Nutritional value per serving
- Calories: 245- Carbs: 35g- Fiber: 9g- Sugars: 7g- Protein: 9g- Saturated fat: 1g
- Unsaturated fat: 3g

Difficulty rating: ★★☆☆☆

36. GRILLED SHRIMP AND MANGO SALAD

Brief Introduction

This Grilled Shrimp and Mango Salad combines succulent grilled shrimp with the sweet, tropical taste of mango, mixed greens, and a zesty lime dressing. It's a refreshing and protein-rich dish that's perfect for a satisfying and nutritious lunch, aligning with the principles of a high-protein, low-fat diet.

Ingredients for 1 serving

- 4 oz shrimp, peeled and deveined
- 1 cup mixed greens
- 1/2 ripe mango, peeled and cubed
- 1/4 avocado, sliced
- 1 tablespoon red onion, finely chopped
- 1 tablespoon cilantro, chopped
- Juice of 1 lime
- 1 teaspoon olive oil
- Salt and pepper to taste

Preparation time and Cooking time

- Preparation time: 10 minutes
- Cooking time: 5 minutes

Directions

1. Preheat the grill to medium-high heat.
2. Season the shrimp with salt and pepper, then grill for 2-3 minutes on each side or until they are pink and opaque.
3. In a large bowl, combine the mixed greens, mango cubes, avocado slices, and chopped red onion.
4. In a small bowl, whisk together the lime juice, olive oil, chopped cilantro, salt, and pepper to create the dressing.
5. Add the grilled shrimp to the salad mixture.
6. Drizzle the dressing over the salad and gently toss to combine.
7. Serve the salad immediately, garnished with additional cilantro if desired.

Nutritional value per serving

- Calories: 300- Carbs: 22g- Fiber: 5g- Sugars: 15g- Protein: 24g- Saturated fat: 1.5g
- Unsaturated fat: 3g

Difficulty rating: ★★☆☆☆

37. CHICKEN AND SPINACH WRAP

Brief Introduction

This Chicken and Spinach Wrap is a delicious, nutritious option for lunch, combining lean protein, fresh vegetables, and whole grains. It's perfectly aligned with a high-protein, low-fat diet, making it an ideal choice for those looking to maintain a healthy lifestyle without sacrificing flavor.

Ingredients for 1 serving

- 3 oz grilled chicken breast, thinly sliced
- 1 whole wheat tortilla (8-inch diameter)
- ¼ cup fresh spinach leaves
- 2 tbsp low-fat Greek yogurt
- 1 tbsp salsa
- ¼ cup diced tomatoes
- ¼ cup shredded carrots
- Salt and pepper to taste

Preparation time and Cooking time

- Preparation time: 10 minutes
- Cooking time: 0 minutes

Directions

1. Lay the whole wheat tortilla flat on a clean surface.
2. Spread the low-fat Greek yogurt evenly over the tortilla.
3. Add the salsa on top of the yogurt.
4. Arrange the grilled chicken slices down the center of the tortilla.
5. Top the chicken with fresh spinach leaves, diced tomatoes, and shredded carrots.
6. Season with salt and pepper to taste.
7. Carefully roll the tortilla, folding in the sides first to enclose the fillings, then rolling from the bottom up tightly.
8. Cut the wrap in half diagonally and serve immediately.

Nutritional value per serving

- Calories: 320- Carbs: 36g- Fiber: 5g- Sugars: 4g- Protein: 28g- Saturated fat: 1g
- Unsaturated fat: 2g

Difficulty rating: ★★☆☆☆

38. TURKEY AND CRANBERRY SALAD

Brief Introduction

Enjoy a refreshing and nutritious Turkey and Cranberry Salad, perfect for a light yet satisfying lunch. This salad combines lean turkey breast with the sweet tang of cranberries and a mix of greens, offering a delightful balance of flavors and textures. It's an excellent choice for those following a high-protein, low-fat diet.

Ingredients for 1 serving

- 3 oz cooked turkey breast, diced
- 1 cup mixed greens (such as spinach, arugula, and romaine)
- 1/4 cup dried cranberries
- 1/4 cup sliced cucumber
- 1/4 cup cherry tomatoes, halved
- 2 tablespoons red onion, thinly sliced
- 1 tablespoon balsamic vinegar
- 1 teaspoon olive oil
- Salt and pepper to taste

Preparation time and Cooking time

- Preparation time: 10 minutes
- Cooking time: 0 minutes

Directions

1. In a large salad bowl, combine the mixed greens, dried cranberries, sliced cucumber, cherry tomatoes, and red onion.
2. Add the diced turkey breast to the salad bowl.
3. In a small bowl, whisk together the balsamic vinegar, olive oil, salt, and pepper to create the dressing.

4. Drizzle the dressing over the salad and toss gently to ensure all ingredients are evenly coated.
5. Serve the salad immediately, or chill in the refrigerator for 10 minutes before serving if a cooler salad is preferred.

Nutritional value per serving

- Calories: 300- Carbs: 34g- Fiber: 4g- Sugars: 24g- Protein: 25g- Saturated fat: 1g
- Unsaturated fat: 2g

Difficulty rating: ★★☆☆☆

39. LENTIL AND VEGGIE BOWL

Brief Introduction

This Lentil and Veggie Bowl is a hearty, nutritious option for lunch, perfectly aligning with a high-protein, low-fat diet. Packed with fiber-rich lentils and a variety of colorful vegetables, it's designed to keep you satisfied and energized throughout your day.

Ingredients for 1 serving

- 1/2 cup cooked lentils
- 1/2 cup broccoli florets, steamed
- 1/4 cup carrots, diced and steamed
- 1/4 cup red bell pepper, diced
- 1/4 cup spinach leaves, raw or slightly wilted
- 1 tablespoon red onion, finely chopped
- 1 teaspoon olive oil
- 1 tablespoon lemon juice
- Salt and pepper to taste
- 1/4 teaspoon garlic powder (optional)

Preparation time and Cooking time

- Preparation time: 10 minutes
- Cooking time: 20 minutes (if starting with uncooked lentils)

Directions

1. If using uncooked lentils, rinse them thoroughly and boil in water according to package instructions until tender. Drain any excess water and set aside.
2. Steam the broccoli florets and diced carrots until they are tender but still crisp, about 5-7 minutes.
3. In a large bowl, combine the cooked lentils, steamed broccoli, steamed carrots, raw red bell pepper, and spinach leaves.
4. Add the finely chopped red onion to the bowl for a sharp, fresh flavor.
5. Drizzle olive oil and lemon juice over the mixture. Season with salt, pepper, and garlic powder (if using). Toss well to ensure all ingredients are evenly coated with the dressing and seasoning.
6. Taste and adjust the seasoning if necessary, adding more salt, pepper, or lemon juice as desired.
7. Serve the lentil and veggie bowl immediately, or chill in the refrigerator for a refreshing cold salad.

Nutritional value per serving

- Calories: 320- Carbs: 45g- Fiber: 15g- Sugars: 4g- Protein: 18g- Saturated fat: 1g
- Unsaturated fat: 2g

Difficulty rating: ★★☆☆☆

40. SPICY CHICKEN AND CUCUMBER SALAD

Brief Introduction

A refreshing, protein-packed dish that brings together tender, seasoned chicken with cool, crisp cucumbers. The subtle heat from the spices perfectly complements the crunch of the cucumber, creating a flavorful yet light meal.

Ingredients for 1 serving

- 4 oz grilled chicken breast, thinly sliced
- 1 cup cucumber, spiralized or thinly sliced
- 1/4 cup red bell pepper, thinly sliced
- 1/4 cup carrot, julienned
- 2 tablespoons red onion, finely chopped
- 1 tablespoon fresh cilantro, chopped
- 1 tablespoon lime juice
- 1/2 tablespoon olive oil
- 1/2 teaspoon chili flakes (adjust to taste)
- Salt and pepper to taste

Preparation time and Cooking time
- Preparation time: 15 minutes
- Cooking time: 0 minutes

Directions
1. In a large mixing bowl, combine the spiralized cucumber, red bell pepper slices, julienned carrot, and chopped red onion.
2. Add the thinly sliced grilled chicken breast to the bowl with the vegetables.
3. In a small bowl, whisk together lime juice, olive oil, chili flakes, salt, and pepper to create the dressing.
4. Pour the dressing over the chicken and vegetable mixture, tossing well to ensure everything is evenly coated.
5. Garnish the salad with chopped fresh cilantro.
6. Serve the salad immediately, or let it chill in the refrigerator for about 10 minutes to enhance the flavors.

Nutritional value per serving
- Calories: 250- Carbs: 10g- Fiber: 2g- Sugars: 5g- Protein: 26g- Saturated fat: 2g
- Unsaturated fat: 3g

Difficulty rating: ★★☆☆☆

CHAPTER 5: DELICIOUS AND BALANCED DINNERS

5.1: SATISFYING AND NUTRITIOUS DINNERS

41. GRILLED LEMON HERB CHICKEN

Brief Introduction

This Grilled Lemon Herb Chicken recipe is a light and flavorful dish that perfectly fits a high-protein, low-fat diet. Marinated in lemon juice and herbs, the chicken is grilled to perfection, offering a satisfying and nutritious dinner option.

Ingredients for 1 serving
- 4 oz chicken breast, boneless and skinless
- 1 tablespoon olive oil
- Juice of 1 lemon
- 1 garlic clove, minced
- 1 teaspoon dried oregano
- 1 teaspoon dried thyme
- Salt and pepper to taste

Preparation time and Cooking time
- Preparation time: 10 minutes (plus at least 30 minutes for marinating)
- Cooking time: 10 minutes

Directions
1. In a small bowl, whisk together olive oil, lemon juice, minced garlic, oregano, thyme, salt, and pepper to create the marinade.
2. Place the chicken breast in a resealable plastic bag or shallow dish and pour the marinade over it. Ensure the chicken is well-coated. Seal or cover and refrigerate for at least 30 minutes, or up to 4 hours for more flavor.
3. Preheat the grill to medium-high heat.
4. Remove the chicken from the marinade, letting excess drip off. Discard the remaining marinade.
5. Grill the chicken for 5 minutes on each side, or until it reaches an internal temperature of 165°F (74°C).
6. Let the chicken rest for a few minutes before slicing or serving whole.

Nutritional value per serving
- Calories: 290- Carbs: 3g- Fiber: 1g- Sugars: 1g- Protein: 26g- Saturated fat: 2g
- Unsaturated fat: 5g

Difficulty rating: ★★☆☆☆

42. BAKED COD WITH ASPARAGUS

Brief introduction

A light, flavorful dish featuring tender, flaky cod paired with roasted asparagus. This simple yet elegant recipe is high in protein and low in calories, making it an ideal option for a healthy lunch or dinner.

Ingredients for 1 serving

- 4 oz cod fillet
- 1 cup asparagus spears, trimmed
- 1 tablespoon olive oil
- 1/4 teaspoon garlic powder
- 1/4 teaspoon paprika
- Salt and pepper to taste
- Lemon wedges for serving

Preparation time and Cooking time

- Preparation time: 5 minutes
- Cooking time: 20 minutes

Directions

1. Preheat the oven to 400°F (200°C).
2. Place the cod fillet and asparagus spears on a baking sheet lined with parchment paper.
3. Drizzle olive oil over the cod and asparagus. Sprinkle garlic powder, paprika, salt, and pepper evenly over the top.
4. Gently toss the asparagus to ensure they are well coated with the seasoning.
5. Bake in the preheated oven for 20 minutes, or until the cod flakes easily with a fork and the asparagus is tender.
6. Serve immediately with lemon wedges on the side for added flavor.

Nutritional value per serving

- Calories: 250- Carbs: 5g- Fiber: 2g- Sugars: 2g- Protein: 23g- Saturated fat: 1g
- Unsaturated fat: 10g

Difficulty rating: ★★☆☆☆

43. TURKEY AND SPINACH STUFFED PEPPERS

Brief Introduction

This Turkey and Spinach Stuffed Peppers recipe is a vibrant, nutritious dinner option that perfectly aligns with a high-protein, low-fat diet. Featuring lean turkey breast, fresh spinach, and bell peppers, it's designed to satisfy your hunger while supporting your health goals.

Ingredients for 1 serving

- 2 large bell peppers, halved and seeded
- 4 oz lean ground turkey
- 1 cup spinach, chopped
- 1/4 cup onion, finely diced
- 1 clove garlic, minced
- 1/2 cup canned diced tomatoes, drained
- 1/4 tsp ground cumin
- 1/4 tsp paprika
- Salt and pepper to taste
- 1/4 cup low-fat shredded cheese (optional)
- Non-stick cooking spray

Preparation time and Cooking time

- Preparation time: 15 minutes
- Cooking time: 25 minutes

Directions

1. Preheat the oven to 375°F (190°C). Prepare a baking dish by lightly spraying it with non-stick cooking spray.
2. Place the bell pepper halves in the baking dish, cut-side up.
3. In a skillet over medium heat, cook the ground turkey, onion, and garlic until the turkey is no longer pink and the onions are translucent, about 5-7 minutes.
4. Add the chopped spinach, diced tomatoes, cumin, paprika, salt, and pepper to the skillet. Cook for an additional 2-3 minutes, or until the spinach is wilted.
5. Spoon the turkey and spinach mixture evenly into the bell pepper halves.
6. If using, sprinkle the low-fat shredded cheese over the top of each stuffed pepper.
7. Cover the baking dish with aluminum foil and bake in the preheated oven for 20 minutes.
8. Remove the foil and bake for an additional 5 minutes, or until the cheese is melted and bubbly.
9. Let the stuffed peppers cool for a few minutes before serving.

Nutritional value per serving

- Calories: 290- Carbs: 18g- Fiber: 5g- Sugars: 10g- Protein: 28g- Saturated fat: 2g
- Unsaturated fat: 3g

Difficulty rating: ★★☆☆☆

44. GRILLED TOFU WITH STEAMED BROCCOLI

Brief Introduction

A nutritious and satisfying plant-based meal, perfect for those seeking a high-protein, low-calorie option. The tofu is grilled to perfection, offering a deliciously crispy texture, while the steamed broccoli adds a dose of vitamins and fiber.

Ingredients for 1 serving

- 1/2 cup firm tofu, pressed and sliced into strips
- 1 cup broccoli florets
- 1 tablespoon low-sodium soy sauce
- 1 teaspoon olive oil
- 1/4 teaspoon garlic powder
- 1/4 teaspoon ground black pepper
- 1/2 teaspoon sesame seeds (for garnish)

Preparation time and Cooking time

- Preparation time: 15 minutes
- Cooking time: 10 minutes

Directions

1. Press the tofu to remove excess moisture by wrapping it in a clean kitchen towel and placing a heavy object on top for at least 10 minutes.
2. Preheat a grill pan over medium heat and brush it with olive oil.
3. In a small bowl, mix the low-sodium soy sauce, garlic powder, and black pepper.
4. Brush the tofu strips with the soy sauce mixture, ensuring all sides are coated.
5. Place the tofu strips on the grill pan and cook for about 3-4 minutes on each side, or until grill marks appear and the tofu is heated through.
6. While the tofu is grilling, steam the broccoli florets until tender but still crisp, about 5-7 minutes.
7. Serve the grilled tofu strips alongside the steamed broccoli. Garnish with sesame seeds.

Nutritional value per serving

- Calories: 200- Carbs: 10g- Fiber: 4g- Sugars: 3g- Protein: 16g- Saturated fat: 1g
- Unsaturated fat: 3g

Difficulty rating: ★★☆☆☆

45. CHICKEN AND ZUCCHINI NOODLES

Brief Introduction

This Chicken and Zucchini Noodles recipe is a light yet satisfying dinner option, perfect for those on a high-protein, low-fat diet. It combines the lean protein of chicken with the low-carb alternative of zucchini noodles, all tossed in a flavorful pesto sauce for a meal that's both nutritious and delicious.

Ingredients for 1 serving

- 4 oz chicken breast, grilled and sliced
- 1 large zucchini, spiralized into noodles
- 2 tbsp homemade or store-bought low-fat pesto sauce
- 1/2 tbsp olive oil
- Salt and pepper to taste
- 1 tbsp grated Parmesan cheese (optional for garnish)
- Fresh basil leaves (optional for garnish)

Preparation time and Cooking time

- Preparation time: 10 minutes
- Cooking time: 15 minutes

Directions

1. Preheat a non-stick skillet over medium heat and add olive oil.
2. Add the spiralized zucchini noodles to the skillet, seasoning with salt and pepper. Sauté for 2-3 minutes until the noodles are tender but still firm.
3. In the meantime, grill the chicken breast until fully cooked, then slice it thinly.
4. Add the grilled chicken slices to the skillet with the zucchini noodles.
5. Lower the heat and add the pesto sauce to the skillet, tossing everything together until the chicken and noodles are well-coated with the pesto.
6. Once heated through, remove from the heat and transfer to a serving plate.
7. Garnish with grated Parmesan cheese and fresh basil leaves if desired.
8. Serve immediately while hot.

Nutritional value per serving

- Calories: 290- Carbs: 6g- Fiber: 2g- Sugars: 4g- Protein: 28g- Saturated fat: 2g
- Unsaturated fat: 5g

Difficulty rating: ★★☆☆☆

46. SHRIMP AND CAULIFLOWER RICE STIR-FRY

Brief Introduction

Enjoy a light and flavorful Shrimp and Cauliflower Rice Stir-Fry, perfect for a nutritious dinner. This dish combines succulent shrimp with aromatic spices and hearty cauliflower rice, creating a satisfying meal that's high in protein and low in both fat and carbs.

Ingredients for 1 serving

- 4 oz shrimp, peeled and deveined
- 1 cup cauliflower rice
- 1/4 cup bell peppers, diced
- 1/4 cup onions, diced
- 1 clove garlic, minced
- 1 tablespoon soy sauce (low sodium)
- 1/2 tablespoon olive oil
- 1/4 teaspoon ginger, grated
- Salt and pepper to taste
- 1 tablespoon green onions, sliced for garnish

Preparation time and Cooking time

- Preparation time: 10 minutes
- Cooking time: 10 minutes

Directions

1. Heat olive oil in a large skillet over medium-high heat.
2. Add the garlic, ginger, bell peppers, and onions to the skillet. Sauté for 2-3 minutes until the vegetables are slightly softened.
3. Increase the heat to high and add the shrimp to the skillet. Season with salt and pepper. Cook for 2-3 minutes, or until the shrimp turn pink and are nearly cooked through.

4. Stir in the cauliflower rice and soy sauce. Mix well to combine all the ingredients. Cook for an additional 3-4 minutes, or until the cauliflower rice is tender and the shrimp are fully cooked.
5. Taste and adjust seasoning if necessary.
6. Garnish with sliced green onions before serving.

Nutritional value per serving

- Calories: 250- Carbs: 14g- Fiber: 3g- Sugars: 5g- Protein: 25g- Saturated fat: 1g
- Unsaturated fat: 3g

Difficulty rating: ★★☆☆☆

47. TURKEY MEATBALLS WITH SPAGHETTI SQUASH

Brief Introduction

This Turkey Meatballs with Spaghetti Squash recipe is a delightful twist on a classic, offering a high-protein, low-fat, and low-sugar dinner option. Perfect for those adhering to a 1200-calorie diet plan, it combines the savory taste of seasoned turkey meatballs with the light, slightly sweet strands of spaghetti squash, making it a nutritious and satisfying meal.

Ingredients for 1 serving

- 1/2 medium spaghetti squash
- 4 oz ground turkey (93% lean)
- 1/4 cup finely chopped onion
- 1 clove garlic, minced
- 1 tablespoon fresh parsley, chopped
- 1/4 teaspoon salt
- 1/4 teaspoon black pepper
- 1/4 teaspoon dried oregano
- 1/4 cup low-sodium marinara sauce
- 1 teaspoon olive oil
- 2 tablespoons grated Parmesan cheese

Preparation time and Cooking time

- Preparation time: 15 minutes
- Cooking time: 45 minutes

Directions

1. Preheat the oven to 400°F (200°C). Line a baking sheet with parchment paper.
2. Cut the spaghetti squash in half lengthwise and scoop out the seeds. Place the squash halves cut-side down on the prepared baking sheet. Bake for 30-40 minutes, or until the flesh is tender and easily shreds with a fork.
3. While the squash is baking, combine the ground turkey, chopped onion, minced garlic, parsley, salt, pepper, and oregano in a bowl. Mix well.
4. Form the turkey mixture into small meatballs, about 1 inch in diameter.
5. Heat olive oil in a non-stick skillet over medium heat. Add the meatballs and cook, turning occasionally, until browned on all sides and cooked through, about 10-12 minutes.
6. Warm the marinara sauce in a small saucepan over low heat.
7. Once the spaghetti squash is cooked, use a fork to scrape the inside to create spaghetti-like strands. Place the strands on a plate.
8. Top the spaghetti squash with the cooked turkey meatballs and marinara sauce.
9. Sprinkle grated Parmesan cheese over the top before serving.

Nutritional value per serving

- Calories: 290- Carbs: 20g- Fiber: 4g- Sugars: 8g- Protein: 28g- Saturated fat: 3g
- Unsaturated fat: 2g

Difficulty rating: ★★☆☆☆

48. GRILLED SALMON WITH GREEN BEANS

Brief Introduction

Enjoy a healthy and flavorful dinner with this Grilled Salmon with Green Beans recipe. Perfectly aligned with a high-protein, low-fat diet, this dish is not only delicious but also packed with essential nutrients, making it an ideal choice for a satisfying and nutritious dinner.

Ingredients for 1 serving

- 4 oz salmon fillet
- 1 cup green beans, trimmed
- 1 teaspoon olive oil
- Salt and pepper to taste
- 1/2 lemon, for juice
- 1 garlic clove, minced
- 1/2 teaspoon dried dill (optional)

Preparation time and Cooking time

- Preparation time: 10 minutes
- Cooking time: 15 minutes

Directions

1. Preheat the grill to medium-high heat.
2. Brush the salmon fillet with 1/2 teaspoon olive oil and season with salt, pepper, and dried dill if using.
3. Toss the green beans with the remaining olive oil, minced garlic, and a pinch of salt and pepper.
4. Place the salmon on the grill, skin-side down, and cook for 6-8 minutes. Flip carefully and grill for another 4-6 minutes, or until the salmon is cooked through and flakes easily with a fork.
5. While the salmon is grilling, place the green beans in a grill basket or on a piece of aluminum foil with holes poked for ventilation. Grill alongside the salmon for about 10 minutes, shaking the basket or stirring occasionally, until the beans are tender and slightly charred.
6. Squeeze fresh lemon juice over the grilled salmon and green beans before serving.

Nutritional value per serving

- Calories: 295- Carbs: 10g- Fiber: 4g- Sugars: 3g- Protein: 23g- Saturated fat: 2g
- Unsaturated fat: 7g

Difficulty rating: ★★☆☆☆

49. CHICKEN AND QUINOA STUFFED BELL PEPPERS

Brief Introduction

This Chicken and Quinoa Stuffed Bell Peppers recipe is a perfect dinner option that combines high-quality protein from chicken, the nutty flavor of quinoa, and the natural sweetness of bell peppers. Designed to fit into a 1200-calorie diet plan, this dish is not only filling but also packed with nutrients, making it an ideal choice for a satisfying and nutritious dinner.

Ingredients for 1 serving

- 2 large bell peppers, halved and seeds removed
- 4 oz chicken breast, cooked and shredded
- 1/2 cup cooked quinoa
- 1/4 cup black beans, rinsed and drained
- 1/4 cup corn kernels (fresh or frozen and thawed)
- 1/4 cup diced tomatoes
- 1/4 cup shredded low-fat cheese
- 1 tablespoon chopped cilantro
- 1 teaspoon cumin
- Salt and pepper to taste
- Cooking spray

Preparation time and Cooking time

- Preparation time: 15 minutes
- Cooking time: 25 minutes

Directions

1. Preheat the oven to 375°F (190°C) and lightly spray a baking dish with cooking spray.
2. In a bowl, mix the shredded chicken, cooked quinoa, black beans, corn, diced tomatoes, cumin, salt, and pepper.
3. Arrange the bell pepper halves in the prepared baking dish, cut-side up.
4. Spoon the chicken and quinoa mixture evenly into each bell pepper half.
5. Cover the baking dish with aluminum foil and bake in the preheated oven for about 20 minutes, or until the peppers are tender.
6. Remove the foil, sprinkle the shredded cheese over each stuffed pepper, and return to the oven, uncovered, for an additional 5 minutes, or until the cheese is melted and bubbly.
7. Garnish with chopped cilantro before serving.

Nutritional value per serving

- Calories: 295- Carbs: 32g- Fiber: 6g- Sugars: 7g- Protein: 28g- Saturated fat: 2g
- Unsaturated fat: 2g

Difficulty rating: ★★☆☆☆

50. BAKED TILAPIA WITH BRUSSELS SPROUTS

Brief Introduction

This Baked Tilapia with Brussels Sprouts recipe is a light, nutritious dinner option that perfectly aligns with a high-protein, low-fat diet. The delicate flavors of tilapia are complemented by the roasted, slightly nutty taste of Brussels sprouts, making for a meal that is as satisfying as it is healthy.

Ingredients for 1 serving

- 4 oz tilapia fillet
- 1 cup Brussels sprouts, halved
- 1 tablespoon olive oil
- 1/2 teaspoon garlic powder
- 1/2 teaspoon paprika
- Salt and pepper to taste
- Lemon wedge for serving

Preparation time and Cooking time

- Preparation time: 10 minutes
- Cooking time: 20 minutes

Directions

1. Preheat the oven to 400°F (200°C).
2. Place the Brussels sprouts on a baking sheet and drizzle with half the olive oil. Sprinkle with salt and pepper to taste. Toss to coat evenly.
3. Bake the Brussels sprouts in the preheated oven for 10 minutes.

4. While the Brussels sprouts are baking, season the tilapia fillet with garlic powder, paprika, salt, and pepper. Drizzle the remaining olive oil over the tilapia.

5. After the Brussels sprouts have cooked for 10 minutes, remove the baking sheet from the oven. Push the Brussels sprouts to one side of the baking sheet, and place the seasoned tilapia fillet on the other side.

6. Return the baking sheet to the oven and bake for an additional 10 minutes, or until the tilapia is flaky and cooked through and the Brussels sprouts are tender and slightly caramelized.

7. Serve the baked tilapia and Brussels sprouts with a lemon wedge on the side for added flavor.

Nutritional value per serving

- Calories: 280- Carbs: 11g- Fiber: 4g- Sugars: 3g- Protein: 25g- Saturated fat: 2g
- Unsaturated fat: 7g

Difficulty rating: ★★☆☆☆

5.2: FAMILY-FRIENDLY MEALS UNDER 300 CALORIES

51. GRILLED CHICKEN AND VEGGIE SKEWERS

Brief Introduction

A flavorful, protein-rich meal that combines tender, seasoned chicken with a colorful variety of grilled vegetables. This easy-to-make dish is both nutritious and satisfying, making it an excellent choice for a light, healthy lunch or dinner.

Ingredients for 1 serving

- 4 oz chicken breast, cut into cubes
- 1/2 bell pepper, cut into pieces
- 1/2 zucchini, sliced
- 1/2 red onion, cut into wedges
- 1 tablespoon olive oil
- 1/2 teaspoon garlic powder
- 1/2 teaspoon dried oregano
- Salt and pepper to taste
- Wooden or metal skewers

Preparation time and Cooking time

- Preparation time: 15 minutes
- Cooking time: 10 minutes

Directions

1. If using wooden skewers, soak them in water for at least 30 minutes to prevent burning.
2. Preheat the grill to medium-high heat.
3. In a large bowl, combine the chicken cubes, bell pepper pieces, zucchini slices, and red onion wedges.
4. Drizzle olive oil over the chicken and vegetables. Add garlic powder, oregano, salt, and pepper. Toss to coat evenly.
5. Thread the chicken and vegetables alternately onto the skewers.
6. Place the skewers on the grill. Cook for 5 minutes, then turn and cook for another 5 minutes or until the chicken is cooked through and the vegetables are slightly charred.
7. Remove from the grill and let rest for a few minutes before serving.

Nutritional value per serving

- Calories: 290- Carbs: 8g- Fiber: 2g- Sugars: 4g- Protein: 26g- Saturated fat: 2g
- Unsaturated fat: 5g

Difficulty rating: ★★☆☆☆

52. SPICY TURKEY LETTUCE WRAPS

Brief Introduction

Enjoy a flavorful and nutritious meal with these Spicy Turkey Lettuce Wraps. Combining lean ground turkey with a blend of spices and wrapped in crisp lettuce leaves, this dish is a perfect example of a high-protein, low-fat, and low-sugar meal that doesn't compromise on taste. Ideal for a family-friendly dinner that everyone will enjoy.

Ingredients for 1 serving

- 4 oz lean ground turkey
- 1/4 tsp chili powder
- 1/4 tsp cumin
- 1/4 tsp garlic powder
- Salt and pepper to taste
- 1/2 cup diced tomatoes
- 1/4 cup diced red onion
- 1/4 cup chopped cilantro
- 4 large lettuce leaves (such as romaine or butter lettuce)
- 1 tbsp low-fat Greek yogurt
- 1 tbsp salsa (optional for extra spice)

Preparation time and Cooking time

- Preparation time: 10 minutes
- Cooking time: 10 minutes

Directions

1. Heat a non-stick skillet over medium heat. Add the ground turkey, chili powder, cumin, garlic powder, salt, and pepper. Cook until the turkey is browned and no longer pink, breaking it into crumbles as it cooks, about 5-7 minutes.
2. Remove the skillet from heat and stir in the diced tomatoes, red onion, and cilantro until well combined.
3. Lay the lettuce leaves on a flat surface, forming cups.
4. Spoon the turkey mixture evenly among the lettuce leaves.
5. Top each wrap with a dollop of low-fat Greek yogurt and a spoonful of salsa if desired for additional spice.
6. Serve immediately while the filling is still warm.

Nutritional value per serving

- Calories: 200- Carbs: 8g- Fiber: 2g- Sugars: 4g- Protein: 22g- Saturated fat: 1g
- Unsaturated fat: 2g

Difficulty rating: ★★☆☆☆

53. LEMON HERB GRILLED SHRIMP

Brief Introduction

A light and flavorful dish, featuring succulent shrimp marinated in a zesty lemon and herb blend. Grilled to perfection, this protein-packed recipe is low in calories and full of fresh, vibrant flavors.

Ingredients for 1 serving

- 6 large shrimp, peeled and deveined
- 1 tablespoon olive oil
- 1 tablespoon lemon juice
- 1/2 teaspoon dried oregano
- 1/2 teaspoon dried thyme
- Salt and pepper to taste
- Lemon wedges for serving

Preparation time and Cooking time

- Preparation time: 10 minutes
- Cooking time: 6 minutes

Directions

1. In a bowl, whisk together olive oil, lemon juice, oregano, thyme, salt, and pepper.
2. Add shrimp to the bowl and toss to coat evenly. Let marinate for 5 to 10 minutes.
3. Preheat a grill or grill pan over medium-high heat.
4. Remove shrimp from the marinade, discarding any excess marinade.
5. Grill shrimp for 2-3 minutes on each side, or until they are pink and opaque.
6. Serve immediately with lemon wedges on the side.

Nutritional value per serving

- Calories: 200- Carbs: 2g- Fiber: 0g- Sugars: 0g- Protein: 24g- Saturated fat: 1g
- Unsaturated fat: 5g

Difficulty rating: ★★☆☆☆

54. CHICKEN AND VEGGIE STIR-FRY

Brief Introduction

A delicious, protein-packed meal that combines tender chicken with a colorful array of fresh vegetables, all cooked in a flavorful, low-calorie sauce. This quick and easy stir-fry is perfect for a healthy lunch or dinner, delivering a satisfying balance of taste and nutrition

Ingredients for 1 serving

- 4 oz chicken breast, thinly sliced
- 1 cup mixed vegetables (broccoli, bell peppers, carrots, and snap peas)
- 1 tablespoon low-sodium soy sauce
- 1 teaspoon sesame oil
- 1 garlic clove, minced

- 1/2 teaspoon ginger, grated
- Non-stick cooking spray
- Salt and pepper to taste

Preparation time and Cooking time

- Preparation time: 10 minutes
- Cooking time: 10 minutes

Directions

1. Heat a large skillet or wok over medium-high heat and coat with non-stick cooking spray.
2. Add the thinly sliced chicken breast to the skillet, season with salt and pepper, and stir-fry until cooked through and no longer pink, about 5-6 minutes. Remove chicken from the skillet and set aside.
3. In the same skillet, add the minced garlic and grated ginger, sautéing for about 30 seconds until fragrant.
4. Add the mixed vegetables to the skillet and stir-fry for 3-4 minutes until they are tender-crisp.
5. Return the cooked chicken to the skillet, add the low-sodium soy sauce and sesame oil, and toss everything together until well combined and heated through.
6. Serve the chicken and veggie stir-fry immediately.

Nutritional value per serving

- Calories: 250- Carbs: 10g- Fiber: 3g- Sugars: 4g- Protein: 26g- Saturated fat: 1g
- Unsaturated fat: 2g

Difficulty rating: ★★☆☆☆

55. TURKEY AND SPINACH STUFFED MUSHROOMS

Brief Introduction

A flavorful and nutritious dish that combines lean, seasoned turkey with sautéed spinach, all packed into savory mushroom caps. This high-protein, low-calorie recipe is perfect for a healthy appetizer or a light meal.

Ingredients for 1 serving

- 4 large mushrooms, stems removed
- 4 oz ground turkey
- 1/2 cup spinach, finely chopped
- 1/4 cup onion, finely diced
- 1 clove garlic, minced
- 1/4 cup low-fat feta cheese, crumbled
- 1 tablespoon olive oil
- Salt and pepper to taste
- 1/4 teaspoon dried oregano

Preparation time and Cooking time

- Preparation time: 15 minutes
- Cooking time: 20 minutes

Directions

1. Preheat the oven to 375°F (190°C) and line a baking sheet with parchment paper.
2. In a skillet over medium heat, heat the olive oil and sauté the onion and garlic until translucent, about 3-4 minutes.
3. Add the ground turkey to the skillet, breaking it apart with a spoon. Cook until no longer pink, about 5-6 minutes.
4. Stir in the spinach, cooking until wilted, approximately 2 minutes. Season with salt, pepper, and dried oregano.
5. Remove the skillet from heat and let the mixture cool slightly. Stir in the crumbled feta cheese.
6. Stuff each mushroom cap generously with the turkey and spinach mixture.
7. Place the stuffed mushrooms on the prepared baking sheet and bake in the preheated oven for 15-20 minutes, or until the mushrooms are tender and the filling is heated through.
8. Serve the turkey and spinach stuffed mushrooms hot.

Nutritional value per serving

- Calories: 290- Carbs: 8g- Fiber: 2g- Sugars: 4g- Protein: 25g- Saturated fat: 3g
- Unsaturated fat: 5g

Difficulty rating: ★★☆☆☆

56. GRILLED TOFU AND VEGGIE KEBABS

Brief Introduction

A vibrant, plant-based meal featuring marinated tofu and a colorful assortment of fresh vegetables, all grilled to perfection. This high-protein, low-calorie dish is ideal for a healthy lunch or dinner.

Ingredients for 1 serving

- 1/2 cup firm tofu, pressed and cubed
- 1/4 cup bell peppers, cut into 1-inch pieces
- 1/4 cup zucchini, cut into 1-inch pieces
- 1/4 cup red onion, cut into 1-inch pieces
- 1 tablespoon low-sodium soy sauce
- 1 teaspoon olive oil
- 1/2 teaspoon garlic powder
- 1/4 teaspoon ground black pepper
- Wooden or metal skewers

Preparation time and Cooking time

- Preparation time: 15 minutes
- Cooking time: 10 minutes

Directions

1. In a large bowl, combine the cubed tofu, bell peppers, zucchini, and red onion.
2. In a small bowl, whisk together the low-sodium soy sauce, olive oil, garlic powder, and ground black pepper to create the marinade.
3. Pour the marinade over the tofu and vegetables, tossing gently to ensure everything is evenly coated. Let marinate for at least 10 minutes.
4. If using wooden skewers, soak them in water for at least 30 minutes to prevent burning.
5. Preheat the grill to medium-high heat.
6. Thread the marinated tofu and vegetables onto the skewers, alternating between tofu and vegetables.
7. Grill the kebabs for about 5 minutes on each side, or until the vegetables are tender and the tofu is slightly charred.

8. Serve the kebabs hot, optionally with extra soy sauce or a dipping sauce of your choice on the side.

Nutritional value per serving

- Calories: 200- Carbs: 15g- Fiber: 3g- Sugars: 5g- Protein: 12g- Saturated fat: 1g
- Unsaturated fat: 3g

Difficulty rating: ★★☆☆☆

57. CHICKEN AND BROCCOLI STIR-FRY

Brief Introduction

Simple yet delicious dish, combining tender, protein-rich chicken with crisp, nutrient-dense broccoli. Cooked in a light, flavorful sauce, this stir-fry offers a satisfying, low-calorie meal that's perfect for lunch or dinner.

Ingredients for 1 serving

- 4 oz chicken breast, thinly sliced
- 1 cup broccoli florets
- 1/2 cup bell peppers, sliced
- 1/4 cup onions, sliced
- 2 cloves garlic, minced
- 1 tablespoon low-sodium soy sauce
- 1 teaspoon sesame oil
- 1/2 teaspoon ground ginger
- Salt and pepper to taste
- Non-stick cooking spray

Preparation time and Cooking time

- Preparation time: 10 minutes
- Cooking time: 10 minutes

Directions

1. Heat a large non-stick skillet or wok over medium-high heat and coat with non-stick cooking spray.
2. Add the chicken slices to the skillet and season with salt and pepper. Stir-fry until the chicken is fully cooked and no longer pink, about 3-4 minutes. Remove the chicken from the skillet and set aside.

3. In the same skillet, add the broccoli florets, bell peppers, and onions. Stir-fry for about 2-3 minutes until the vegetables are tender yet crisp.

4. Add the minced garlic to the skillet and stir-fry for an additional 30 seconds until fragrant.

5. Return the cooked chicken to the skillet. Pour in the low-sodium soy sauce, sesame oil, and ground ginger. Stir well to combine all the ingredients.

6. Cook for another 2 minutes, stirring frequently, until everything is heated through and coated in the sauce.

7. Taste and adjust seasoning with additional salt and pepper if needed.

Nutritional value per serving

- Calories: 280- Carbs: 15g- Fiber: 3g- Sugars: 5g- Protein: 26g- Saturated fat: 1g
- Unsaturated fat: 2g

Difficulty rating: ★★☆☆☆

58. TURKEY AND VEGGIE STUFFED ZUCCHINI BOATS

Brief Introduction

Enjoy a wholesome and satisfying dinner with these Turkey and Veggie Stuffed Zucchini Boats. This recipe is a fantastic way to incorporate lean protein and a variety of vegetables into your meal, making it a perfect fit for a high-protein, low-fat diet. It's family-friendly and sure to be a hit with both adults and kids alike.

Ingredients for 1 serving

- 2 medium zucchini, halved lengthwise
- 4 oz lean ground turkey
- 1/4 cup bell peppers, finely diced
- 1/4 cup onions, finely diced
- 1 clove garlic, minced
- 1/2 cup canned diced tomatoes, drained
- 1/4 tsp dried oregano
- 1/4 tsp dried basil
- Salt and pepper to taste
- 1/4 cup low-fat shredded mozzarella cheese
- 1 tbsp olive oil

Preparation time and Cooking time

- Preparation time: 15 minutes
- Cooking time: 25 minutes

Directions

1. Preheat the oven to 375°F (190°C).

2. Scoop out the center of each zucchini half to create a boat, leaving about 1/4 inch of zucchini along the sides. Chop the scooped-out zucchini flesh and set aside.

3. Heat olive oil in a skillet over medium heat. Add the onions, bell peppers, and minced garlic, sautéing until softened, about 3-4 minutes.

4. Add the ground turkey to the skillet, breaking it apart with a spoon. Cook until no longer pink, about 5-6 minutes.

5. Stir in the chopped zucchini flesh, diced tomatoes, oregano, basil, salt, and pepper. Cook for an additional 2-3 minutes.

6. Place the zucchini boats in a baking dish. Spoon the turkey and veggie mixture evenly into each zucchini boat.

7. Sprinkle the low-fat shredded mozzarella cheese over the top of each stuffed zucchini.

8. Bake in the preheated oven for 20 minutes, or until the zucchini is tender and the cheese is melted and slightly golden.

9. Serve hot.

Nutritional value per serving

- Calories: 290- Carbs: 18g- Fiber: 5g- Sugars: 10g- Protein: 28g- Saturated fat: 3g
- Unsaturated fat: 5g

Difficulty rating: ★★☆☆☆

59. GRILLED LEMON HERB SHRIMP

Brief Introduction

Light and refreshing dish featuring succulent shrimp marinated in a zesty blend of lemon and fresh herbs. Grilled to perfection, this high-protein, low-calorie recipe is bursting with flavor and perfect for a quick and healthy meal.

Ingredients for 1 serving

- 6 large shrimp, peeled and deveined
- 1 tablespoon olive oil
- 1 tablespoon lemon juice
- 1/2 teaspoon dried oregano
- 1/2 teaspoon dried thyme
- 1 clove garlic, minced
- Salt and pepper to taste
- Lemon wedges for serving

Preparation time and Cooking time

- Preparation time: 10 minutes
- Cooking time: 6 minutes

Directions

1. In a bowl, combine olive oil, lemon juice, oregano, thyme, minced garlic, salt, and pepper. Mix well to create the marinade.
2. Add the shrimp to the marinade, ensuring each piece is well-coated. Cover and let marinate in the refrigerator for at least 30 minutes.
3. Preheat the grill to medium-high heat.
4. Thread the marinated shrimp onto skewers.
5. Grill the shrimp for 2-3 minutes on each side, or until they turn pink and opaque.
6. Serve the grilled shrimp with additional lemon wedges on the side.

Nutritional value per serving

- Calories: 200- Carbs: 2g- Fiber: 0g- Sugars: 0g- Protein: 24g- Saturated fat: 1g
- Unsaturated fat: 5g

Difficulty rating: ★★☆☆☆

60. CHICKEN AND VEGGIE LETTUCE WRAPS

Brief Introduction

Light, flavorful dish featuring seasoned chicken and fresh vegetables wrapped in crisp lettuce leaves. This low-calorie, high-protein meal offers a refreshing and satisfying way to enjoy a healthy lunch or dinner

Ingredients for 1 serving

- 2 large lettuce leaves (such as Romaine or Bibb lettuce)
- 4 oz chicken breast, grilled and thinly sliced
- 1/4 cup shredded carrots
- 1/4 cup sliced red bell pepper
- 1/4 cup cucumber, sliced into thin strips
- 2 tablespoons low-fat Greek yogurt
- 1 tablespoon fresh cilantro, chopped
- 1 teaspoon lime juice
- Salt and pepper to taste

Preparation time and Cooking time

- Preparation time: 15 minutes
- Cooking time: 10 minutes

Directions

1. Grill the chicken breast seasoned with salt and pepper until fully cooked, then let it cool before slicing thinly.
2. Wash and dry the lettuce leaves carefully to maintain their shape.
3. In a small bowl, mix the Greek yogurt with lime juice, chopped cilantro, and a pinch of salt and pepper to create a dressing.
4. Lay the lettuce leaves flat on a plate or working surface.
5. Place an equal amount of sliced chicken, shredded carrots, sliced red bell pepper, and cucumber strips in the center of each lettuce leaf.
6. Drizzle the Greek yogurt dressing over the filling of each lettuce wrap.
7. Carefully fold the lettuce leaves to enclose the fillings, securing with a toothpick if necessary.
8. Serve immediately to enjoy the crunch of the fresh vegetables with the tender grilled chicken.

Nutritional value per serving

- Calories: 200- Carbs: 8g- Fiber: 2g- Sugars: 4g- Protein: 26g- Saturated fat: 1g
- Unsaturated fat: 2g

Difficulty rating: ★★☆☆☆

CHAPTER 6: GUILT-FREE DESSERTS

6.1: INDULGENT DESSERTS

61. HIGH-PROTEIN CHOCOLATE MOUSSE

Brief Introduction

Rich and indulgent dessert that satisfies your sweet tooth while staying within your nutritional goals. Made with high-protein ingredients and low in sugar, this guilt-free treat is perfect for those looking to enjoy a dessert without derailing their diet.

Ingredients for 1 serving

- 1/2 cup low-fat cottage cheese
- 2 tablespoons unsweetened cocoa powder
- 1 tablespoon erythritol
- 1/2 teaspoon vanilla extract
- A pinch of salt
- 2 tablespoons whipped cream (for topping, optional)
- A few raspberries or strawberries (for garnish, optional)

Preparation time and Cooking time

- Preparation time: 10 minutes
- Cooking time: 0 minutes

Directions

1. Place the low-fat cottage cheese in a blender or food processor.
2. Add the unsweetened cocoa powder, stevia or agave syrup, vanilla extract, and a pinch of salt to the blender.
3. Blend on high until the mixture is completely smooth and creamy, scraping down the sides as needed. This may take a few minutes to achieve a mousse-like consistency.
4. Taste the mixture and adjust sweetness if necessary by adding a little more stevia or agave syrup.
5. Transfer the chocolate mousse to a serving bowl or glass.
6. If desired, top with whipped cream and garnish with raspberries or strawberries for added flavor and presentation.
7. Chill in the refrigerator for at least 1 hour before serving to allow the mousse to set and flavors to meld.

Nutritional value per serving

- Calories: 160- Carbs: 20g- Fiber: 3g- Sugars: 15g- Protein: 16g- Saturated fat: 0.5g
- Unsaturated fat: 1g

Difficulty rating: ★★☆☆☆

62. GREEK YOGURT AND BERRY PARFAIT

Brief Introduction

Nutrient-packed treat that layers creamy Greek yogurt with antioxidant-rich berries. This high-protein, low-sugar option is perfect for a healthy breakfast, snack, or dessert.

Ingredients for 1 serving

- 1/2 cup low-fat Greek yogurt
- 1/4 cup mixed berries (strawberries, blueberries, raspberries)
- 1 tablespoon granola
- 1 teaspoon erythritol

- A pinch of cinnamon (optional)

Preparation time and Cooking time

- Preparation time: 5 minutes
- Cooking time: 0 minutes

Directions

1. In a serving glass or bowl, layer 1/4 cup of low-fat Greek yogurt.
2. Add half of the mixed berries over the yogurt.
3. Sprinkle half of the granola over the berries.
4. Drizzle half of the teaspoon of stevia over the granola.
5. Repeat the layers starting with the remaining Greek yogurt, followed by the remaining berries, granola, and stevia.
6. Optionally, sprinkle a pinch of cinnamon on top for added flavor.
7. Serve immediately or chill in the refrigerator for up to an hour before serving.

Nutritional value per serving
- Calories: 160- Carbs: 20g- Fiber: 5g- Sugars: 10g- Protein: 12g- Saturated fat: 0.5g
- Unsaturated fat: 0g

Difficulty rating: ★☆☆☆☆

63. PROTEIN-PACKED PEANUT BUTTER COOKIES

Brief Introduction

Delicious and nutritious twist on a classic treat. Made with high-protein ingredients and low in sugar, these cookies offer a satisfying, guilt-free snack that supports your diet goals.

Ingredients for 1 serving

- 1/4 cup natural peanut butter
- 1 scoop vanilla protein powder
- 1 tablespoon almond flour
- 1 egg white
- 1/4 teaspoon baking powder
- 1/2 teaspoon vanilla extract
- 2 tablespoons erythritol (or sweetener of choice)

- Pinch of salt

Preparation time and Cooking time

- Preparation time: 10 minutes
- Cooking time: 10 minutes

Directions

1. Preheat your oven to 350°F (175°C) and line a baking sheet with parchment paper.
2. In a mixing bowl, combine the peanut butter, vanilla protein powder, almond flour, egg white, baking powder, vanilla extract, erythritol, and a pinch of salt. Stir until well combined and a dough forms.
3. Divide the dough into 6 equal portions and roll each into a ball. Place the balls on the prepared baking sheet and gently flatten with the back of a fork to create a crisscross pattern.
4. Bake in the preheated oven for 8-10 minutes, or until the edges are slightly golden.
5. Allow the cookies to cool on the baking sheet for 5 minutes before transferring them to a wire rack to cool completely.

Nutritional value per serving

- Calories: 180- Carbs: 8g- Fiber: 2g- Sugars: 1g- Protein: 12g- Saturated fat: 2g
- Unsaturated fat: 4g

Difficulty rating: ★★☆☆☆

64. LOW-FAT RICOTTA AND BERRY TART

Brief Introduction

light, creamy dessert that combines the smoothness of ricotta with the natural sweetness of fresh berries. This guilt-free treat is low in fat and sugar, making it a perfect option for those looking to indulge without compromising their diet.

Ingredients for 1 serving

- 1/2 cup low-fat ricotta cheese
- 1/4 cup mixed berries (strawberries, blueberries, raspberries)

- 1 whole-wheat tart shell (pre-baked)
- 1 tablespoon erythritol
- 1/4 teaspoon vanilla extract
- A pinch of lemon zest
- Mint leaves for garnish

Preparation time and Cooking time

- Preparation time: 10 minutes
- Cooking time: 0 minutes

Directions

1. In a mixing bowl, combine low-fat ricotta cheese, stevia, vanilla extract, and lemon zest. Stir until the mixture is smooth and well combined.
2. Gently fold in the mixed berries, being careful not to crush them.
3. Spoon the ricotta and berry mixture into the pre-baked whole-wheat tart shell, spreading it evenly.
4. Refrigerate the tart for at least 30 minutes to allow the filling to set.
5. Before serving, garnish with mint leaves for a fresh touch.

Nutritional value per serving

- Calories: 160- Carbs: 20g- Fiber: 4g- Sugars: 12g- Protein: 12g- Saturated fat: 1g
- Unsaturated fat: 2g

Difficulty rating: ★★☆☆☆

65. ALMOND FLOUR PROTEIN BROWNIES

Brief Introduction

Indulge in a guilt-free dessert with these Almond Flour Protein Brownies. Crafted to align with Dr. Nowzaradan's dietary principles, these brownies offer a high-protein, low-fat, and low-sugar alternative to traditional treats. Perfect for satisfying your sweet tooth without derailing your diet goals.

Ingredients for 1 serving

- 1/4 cup almond flour

- 1 scoop vanilla or chocolate protein powder
- 1 tbsp unsweetened cocoa powder
- 1/4 tsp baking powder
- A pinch of salt
- 2 tbsp unsweetened almond milk
- 1 egg white
- 1/4 tsp vanilla extract
- 1 tbsp zero-calorie sweetener (e.g., stevia or erythritol)
- Non-stick cooking spray

Preparation time and Cooking time

- Preparation time: 5 minutes
- Cooking time: 12-15 minutes

Directions

1. Preheat your oven to 350°F (175°C). Lightly spray a small baking dish with non-stick cooking spray.
2. In a mixing bowl, combine almond flour, protein powder, unsweetened cocoa powder, baking powder, and a pinch of salt.
3. Add unsweetened almond milk, egg white, vanilla extract, and zero-calorie sweetener to the dry ingredients. Mix until well combined into a smooth batter.
4. Pour the batter into the prepared baking dish, spreading it evenly.
5. Bake in the preheated oven for 12-15 minutes, or until a toothpick inserted into the center comes out clean.
6. Allow the brownie to cool for a few minutes before cutting into portions.

Nutritional value per serving

- Calories: 180- Carbs: 8g- Fiber: 3g- Sugars: 1g- Protein: 16g- Saturated fat: 0.5g
- Unsaturated fat: 3g

Difficulty rating: ★★☆☆☆

66. VANILLA PROTEIN PUDDING

Brief Introduction

Indulge in a creamy and satisfying Vanilla Protein Pudding that perfectly fits your high-protein, low-fat diet. This dessert is not only delicious but also a great way to satisfy your sweet tooth without derailing your nutritional goals. With a rich vanilla flavor and a smooth, pudding-like texture, it's an ideal treat for any time of the day.

Ingredients for 1 serving

- 1 scoop vanilla protein powder
- 1/2 cup unsweetened almond milk
- 1/4 cup Greek yogurt, low-fat
- 1 tsp vanilla extract
- 1/2 tbsp chia seeds
- Stevia to taste

Preparation time and Cooking time

- Preparation time: 5 minutes
- Cooking time: 0 minutes (requires at least 1 hour to chill)

Directions

1. In a mixing bowl, whisk together the vanilla protein powder and unsweetened almond milk until smooth and well combined.
2. Add the Greek yogurt and vanilla extract to the mixture, continuing to whisk until the mixture is smooth.
3. Stir in the chia seeds and sweetener, adjusting the sweetener to taste.
4. Pour the mixture into a serving dish or a mason jar.
5. Cover and refrigerate for at least 1 hour, or until the pudding has set and reached a thick, creamy consistency.
6. Before serving, give the pudding a quick stir to ensure the texture is uniform. Optionally, garnish with a sprinkle of cinnamon or fresh berries.

Nutritional value per serving

- Calories: 180- Carbs: 8g- Fiber: 3g- Sugars: 2g- Protein: 25g- Saturated fat: 0.5g
- Unsaturated fat: 1g

Difficulty rating: ★☆☆☆☆

67 STRAWBERRY ALMOND COTTAGE CHEESE BLISS

Brief Introduction

This refreshing and nutritious dish combines the creamy texture of low-fat cottage cheese with the sweetness of fresh strawberries and the crunch of sliced almonds. Perfect as a light dessert or a satisfying snack, this recipe is not only quick to prepare but also aligns with Dr. Nowzaradan's 1200-calorie diet plan, making it an ideal choice for those looking to lose weight while enjoying delicious flavors

Ingredients for 1 serving

- 1/2 cup low-fat cottage cheese
- 1/2 cup fresh strawberries, diced
- 1 tablespoon sliced almonds

Preparation time and Cooking time

- Preparation time: 5 minutes
- Cooking time: 0 minutes

Directions

1. Place the low-fat cottage cheese in a serving bowl.
2. Top the cottage cheese with diced fresh strawberries.
3. Sprinkle sliced almonds over the strawberries.
4. Gently mix before serving to combine the flavors or layer beautifully to serve as a delightful dessert.

Nutritional value per serving

- Calories: 165- Carbs: 20g- Fiber: 2g- Sugars: 14g - Protein: 14g- Saturated fat: 0.5g
- Unsaturated fat: 2g

Difficulty rating: ★☆☆☆☆

68. PROTEIN-PACKED LEMON CHEESECAKE BITES

Brief Introduction

Indulge in the delightful taste of Protein-Packed Lemon Cheesecake Bites, a guilt-free dessert that perfectly aligns with your health goals. These bites offer a zesty lemon flavor combined with the creamy texture of cheesecake, all while being high in protein and low in both fat and sugar. Ideal for satisfying your sweet tooth without derailing your diet.

Ingredients for 1 serving

- 1/2 cup low-fat Greek yogurt
- 2 tablespoons low-fat cream cheese
- 1 tablespoon vanilla protein powder
- 1 tablespoon lemon juice
- 1 teaspoon lemon zest
- 1 tablespoon almond flour
- 1 tablespoon erythritol (or Stevia)
- Non-stick cooking spray

Preparation time and Cooking time

- Preparation time: 10 minutes
- Cooking time: 0 minutes (requires 1 hour to chill)

Directions

1. In a mixing bowl, combine low-fat Greek yogurt, low-fat cream cheese, vanilla protein powder, lemon juice, and lemon zest. Mix until smooth and well combined.
2. In a separate small bowl, mix almond flour with erythritol.
3. Line a mini muffin pan with mini muffin liners and lightly spray each with non-stick cooking spray.
4. Spoon a small amount of the almond flour mixture into the bottom of each muffin liner, pressing down to form a base.
5. Divide the Greek yogurt mixture among the muffin liners, filling each to the top.
6. Place the mini muffin pan in the freezer and chill for at least 1 hour, or until the cheesecake bites are set.
7. Once set, gently remove the cheesecake bites from the muffin liners and serve immediately.

Nutritional value per serving

- Calories: 180- Carbs: 8g- Fiber: 1g- Sugars: 4g- Protein: 20g- Saturated fat: 1g
- Unsaturated fat: 1g

Difficulty rating: ★★☆☆☆

69. HIGH-PROTEIN APPLE CINNAMON MUFFINS

Brief Introduction

Delicious and nutritious way to enjoy a sweet snack or a quick breakfast. Packed with protein and fiber, these muffins will keep you full and energized without derailing your diet.

Ingredients for 1 serving

- 1 cup oat flour
- 1 scoop vanilla protein powder
- 1/2 teaspoon baking powder
- 1/2 teaspoon baking soda
- 1/4 teaspoon cinnamon
- 1/4 teaspoon salt
- 1/4 cup unsweetened applesauce
- 1/4 cup unsweetened almond milk
- 1/4 teaspoon vanilla extract
- 1/4 cup Stevia or erythritol (or other low-calorie sweeteners)
- 1 medium apple, diced
- 2 large egg whites

Preparation time and Cooking time

- Preparation time: 10 minutes
- Cooking time: 20 minutes

Directions

1. Preheat your oven to 350°F (175°C) and prepare a muffin tin by lightly spraying it with cooking spray.
2. In a large bowl, mix together the oat flour, protein powder, baking powder, baking soda, cinnamon, and salt.

3. In another bowl, whisk together the applesauce, almond milk, vanilla extract, Stevia, and egg whites until smooth.

4. Add the wet ingredients to the dry ingredients and mix until just combined. Fold in the diced apple.

5. Pour the batter into the muffin liners, filling each about 3/4 full.

6. Bake for 20 minutes, or until a toothpick inserted into the center of a muffin comes out clean.

7. Allow the muffins to cool in the pan for 5 minutes before transferring them to a wire rack to cool completely.

Nutritional value per serving

- Calories: 160- Carbs: 12g- Fiber: 3g- Sugars: 3g- Protein: 10g- Saturated fat: 1g
- Unsaturated fat: 2g

Difficulty rating: ★★☆☆☆

70. LOW-FAT CHOCOLATE PROTEIN BARS

Brief Introduction

Indulging in a sweet treat while sticking to a low-calorie diet can be a challenge, but these Low-Fat Chocolate Protein Bars make it easy to satisfy your cravings without derailing your weight loss journey. Packed with high-quality protein and wholesome ingredients, these bars are not only delicious but also provide a nutritious boost to your day.

Ingredients for 1 serving
- 1 scoop chocolate protein powder
- 2 tbsp almond flour
- 1 tbsp unsweetened cocoa powder
- 1/4 cup unsweetened almond milk
- 1 tbsp almond butter
- 1/4 tsp vanilla extract
- A pinch of salt
- Non-stick cooking spray

Preparation time and Cooking time
- Preparation time: 10 minutes
- Cooking time: 0 minutes
- Freezing time: 1 hour

Directions

1. In a mixing bowl, combine the chocolate protein powder, almond flour, unsweetened cocoa powder, and a pinch of salt.

2. Add the unsweetened almond milk, almond butter, and vanilla extract to the dry ingredients. Stir until the mixture is well combined and forms a thick dough.

3. Line a small baking dish or tray with parchment paper and lightly spray with non-stick cooking spray.

4. Press the dough evenly into the prepared dish or tray.

5. Place the dish or tray in the freezer and freeze for at least 1 hour, or until the mixture is solid.

6. Once solid, remove from the freezer and cut into bars.

7. Store the protein bars in an airtight container in the refrigerator or freezer until ready to eat.

Nutritional value per serving

- Calories: 180- Carbs: 8g- Fiber: 3g- Sugars: 1g- Protein: 20g- Saturated fat: 1g
- Unsaturated fat: 3g

Difficulty rating: ★★☆☆☆

6.2: SATISFYING YOUR SWEET TOOTH

71. HIGH-PROTEIN CHOCOLATE CHIP COOKIES

Brief Introduction

With easy-to-find ingredients and a quick preparation process, you can relish a guilt-free dessert that aligns with your health objectives.

Ingredients for 1 serving

- 1 scoop vanilla or chocolate protein powder
- 2 tablespoons almond flour
- 1 tablespoon unsweetened cocoa powder
- 1/4 teaspoon baking powder
- A pinch of salt
- 2 tablespoons unsweetened almond milk
- 1 egg white
- 1/4 teaspoon vanilla extract
- 1 tablespoon zero-calorie sweetener (e.g., stevia or erythritol)
- 2 tablespoons sugar-free chocolate chips

Preparation time and Cooking time

- Preparation time: 10 minutes
- Cooking time: 10 minutes

Directions

1. Preheat your oven to 350°F (175°C) and line a baking sheet with parchment paper.
2. In a mixing bowl, combine protein powder, almond flour, unsweetened cocoa powder, baking powder, and a pinch of salt.
3. Add unsweetened almond milk, egg white, vanilla extract, and zero-calorie sweetener to the dry ingredients. Mix until well combined into a smooth batter.
4. Fold in the sugar-free chocolate chips gently into the batter.
5. Drop tablespoon-sized portions of the batter onto the prepared baking sheet, spacing them about 2 inches apart.

6. Bake in the preheated oven for 8-10 minutes, or until the edges are set but the centers are still soft.
7. Allow the cookies to cool on the baking sheet for 5 minutes before transferring them to a wire rack to cool completely.

Nutritional value per serving
- Calories: 180- Carbs: 10g- Fiber: 3g - Sugars: 1g- Protein: 20g- Saturated fat: 1g
- Unsaturated fat: 2g

Difficulty rating: ★★☆☆☆

72. VANILLA PROTEIN ICE CREAM

Brief Introduction

Indulge in a creamy and refreshing Vanilla Protein Ice Cream, a perfect guilt-free treat to satisfy your sweet cravings while adhering to a high-protein, low-fat diet. This homemade ice cream is not only delicious but also packed with protein, making it an ideal dessert for those looking to maintain a healthy lifestyle without sacrificing taste.

Ingredients for 1 serving

- 1 scoop vanilla protein powder
- 1/2 cup unsweetened almond milk
- 1/4 cup Greek yogurt, low-fat
- 1 tsp vanilla extract
- 1 tbsp zero-calorie sweetener (e.g., stevia or erythritol)
- A pinch of salt
- Ice cubes (as needed for texture)

Preparation time and Cooking time

- Preparation time: 5 minutes
- Freezing time: 2 hours or until firm

Directions

1. In a blender, combine vanilla protein powder, unsweetened almond milk, low-fat Greek yogurt, vanilla extract, zero-calorie sweetener, and a pinch of salt. Blend until the mixture is smooth.
2. Gradually add ice cubes to the blender, blending after each addition, until the mixture reaches your desired ice cream consistency.
3. Transfer the mixture to a freezer-safe container and smooth the top with a spatula.
4. Freeze for at least 2 hours, or until the ice cream is firm.
5. Before serving, let the ice cream sit at room temperature for a few minutes to soften slightly for easier scooping.
6. Serve in a bowl or cone as desired.

Nutritional value per serving

- Calories: 180- Carbs: 8g- Fiber: 1g- Sugars: 4g- Protein: 25g- Saturated fat: 0.5g
- Unsaturated fat: 1g

Difficulty rating: ★★☆☆☆

73. STRAWBERRY PROTEIN SMOOTHIE BOWL

Brief Introduction

Smoothie bowls are a delightful way to start your day, combining nutrition with a burst of flavor. The Strawberry Protein Smoothie Bowl is not only visually appealing but also packed with essential nutrients to fuel your body.

Ingredients for 1 serving

- 1/2 cup unsweetened almond milk
- 1/2 cup frozen strawberries
- 1 scoop vanilla protein powder
- 1/4 cup Greek yogurt, low-fat
- 1 tablespoon chia seeds
- 1/4 teaspoon vanilla extract
- Fresh strawberries for garnish
- A few mint leaves for garnish (optional)

Preparation time and Cooking time

- Preparation time: 5 minutes
- Cooking time: 0 minutes

Directions

1. Place the unsweetened almond milk, frozen strawberries, vanilla protein powder, low-fat Greek yogurt, chia seeds, and vanilla extract into a blender.
2. Blend on high until the mixture is smooth and creamy.
3. Pour the smoothie mixture into a bowl.
4. Garnish with fresh strawberry slices and mint leaves, if using.
5. Serve immediately.

Nutritional value per serving

- Calories: 180- Carbs: 15g- Fiber: 4g- Sugars: 7g- Protein: 20g- Saturated fat: 0.5g
- Unsaturated fat: 1g

Difficulty rating: ★☆☆☆☆

74. CHOCOLATE PROTEIN MUG CAKE

Brief Introduction

The Chocolate Protein Mug Cake is a perfect example of how you can satisfy your chocolate cravings without compromising your health. This quick and easy recipe is not only low in carbs and fats but also packed with protein, making it an ideal choice for a nutritious snack or dessert.

Ingredients for 1 serving
- 1 scoop chocolate protein powder
- 2 tbsp almond flour
- 1 tbsp unsweetened cocoa powder
- 1/4 tsp baking powder
- A pinch of salt
- 1/4 cup unsweetened almond milk
- 1/2 tsp vanilla extract
- Sweetener to taste (e.g., stevia, erythritol)

Preparation time and Cooking time
- Preparation time: 5 minutes
- Cooking time: 1 minute

Directions

1. In a microwave-safe mug, mix together the chocolate protein powder, almond flour, unsweetened cocoa powder, baking powder, and a pinch of salt.
2. Stir in the unsweetened almond milk, vanilla extract, and sweetener until the mixture is smooth and well combined.
3. Microwave on high for 60 seconds, or until the cake rises and sets. Microwave times may vary, so start checking at 45 seconds to prevent overcooking.
4. Let the mug cake cool for a few minutes before eating. Optionally, top with a dollop of low-fat Greek yogurt or fresh berries for extra flavor.

Nutritional value per serving
- Calories: 180- Carbs: 8g- Fiber: 3g- Sugars: 1g- Protein: 20g- Saturated fat: 1g
- Unsaturated fat: 3g

Difficulty rating: ★★☆☆☆

75. BLUEBERRY PROTEIN MUFFINS

Brief Introduction

These muffins are not only easy to prepare but also packed with protein and low in carbs, making them an ideal choice for anyone looking to maintain a healthy lifestyle without sacrificing flavor.

Ingredients for 1 serving

- 1/2 cup almond flour
- 1 scoop vanilla protein powder
- 1/4 cup fresh blueberries
- 1 egg
- 1/4 cup unsweetened almond milk
- 1 tbsp zero-calorie sweetener (e.g., erythritol or stevia)
- 1/2 tsp baking powder
- 1/4 tsp vanilla extract
- Pinch of salt
- Non-stick cooking spray

Preparation time and Cooking time

- Preparation time: 10 minutes

- Cooking time: 20 minutes

Directions

1. Preheat your oven to 350°F (175°C) and prepare a muffin tin by spraying it with non-stick cooking spray or lining it with muffin liners.
2. In a mixing bowl, combine almond flour, vanilla protein powder, baking powder, and a pinch of salt.
3. In another bowl, whisk together the egg, unsweetened almond milk, vanilla extract, and zero-calorie sweetener until well combined.
4. Gradually add the wet ingredients to the dry ingredients, stirring until just combined.
5. Gently fold in the fresh blueberries, being careful not to crush them.
6. Divide the batter evenly among the muffin tin cups, filling each about three-quarters full.
7. Bake in the preheated oven for 20 minutes, or until a toothpick inserted into the center of a muffin comes out clean.
8. Allow the muffins to cool in the pan for 5 minutes before transferring them to a wire rack to cool completely.

Nutritional value per serving
- Calories: 180- Carbs: 10g- Fiber: 3g- Sugars: 2g- Protein: 10g- Saturated fat: 1g
- Unsaturated fat: 3g

Difficulty rating: ★★☆☆☆

76. PEANUT BUTTER PROTEIN BALLS

Brief Introduction

Indulge in these Peanut Butter Protein Balls for a delicious and nutritious snack that perfectly aligns with your health goals. Packed with protein and flavored with natural peanut butter, these bites are an ideal choice for a quick energy boost or a post-workout treat.

Ingredients for 1 serving

- 2 tablespoons natural peanut butter
- 1 scoop vanilla protein powder
- 1 tablespoon ground flaxseed

- 1 tablespoon almond flour
- 2 teaspoons stevia or agave syrup
- A pinch of salt
- 1 tablespoon unsweetened almond milk (adjust as needed for consistency)
- Optional: 1 tablespoon mini dark chocolate chips (ensure to account for added calories)

Preparation time and Cooking time

- Preparation time: 10 minutes
- Cooking time: 0 minutes

Directions

1. In a medium mixing bowl, combine peanut butter, vanilla protein powder, ground flaxseed, almond flour, stevia, and a pinch of salt. Mix until well combined.
2. Gradually add almond milk, one teaspoon at a time, until the mixture reaches a pliable consistency that can be rolled into balls. If using, fold in mini dark chocolate chips.
3. Using your hands, roll the mixture into small balls, about 1 inch in diameter. Place the balls on a plate or baking sheet lined with parchment paper.
4. Refrigerate the protein balls for at least 30 minutes to set.
5. Once set, the Peanut Butter Protein Balls can be stored in an airtight container in the refrigerator for up to a week.

Nutritional value per serving

- Calories: 180- Carbs: 8g- Fiber: 2g- Sugars: 4g- Protein: 10g- Saturated fat: 1g
- Unsaturated fat: 3g

Difficulty rating: ★★☆☆☆

77. LEMON PROTEIN BARS

Brief Introduction

These bars not only satisfy your sweet tooth but also provide a substantial protein boost, making them an ideal snack for those on a weight loss journey. With their refreshing lemon flavor and simple preparation, they are a convenient option for anyone looking to maintain a healthy lifestyle while enjoying delicious food.

Ingredients for 1 serving
- 1 scoop vanilla protein powder
- 1/4 cup almond flour
- 2 tbsp lemon juice
- Zest of 1 lemon
- 1/4 cup unsweetened almond milk
- 1 tbsp olive oil, melted
- 1 tbsp erythritol or another zero-calorie sweetener
- Non-stick cooking spray

Preparation time and Cooking time

- Preparation time: 10 minutes
- Cooking time: 0 minutes
- Freezing time: 2 hours

Directions

1. In a mixing bowl, combine vanilla protein powder, almond flour, lemon zest, and erythritol.
2. Stir in lemon juice, unsweetened almond milk, and melted olive oil until the mixture is well combined and forms a thick dough.
3. Line a small tray or plate with parchment paper and lightly spray with non-stick cooking spray.
4. Press the dough into the prepared tray, forming a uniform layer about 1/2 inch thick.
5. Place the tray in the freezer and freeze for at least 2 hours, or until the mixture is solid.
6. Once solid, remove from the freezer and cut into bars or squares.
7. Store the lemon protein bars in an airtight container in the freezer or refrigerator until ready to serve.

Nutritional value per serving
- Calories: 180- Carbs: 8g- Fiber: 3g- Sugars: 2g- Protein: 20g- Saturated fat: 3g
- Unsaturated fat: 2g

Difficulty rating: ★★☆☆☆

78. CINNAMON PROTEIN DONUTS

Brief Introduction

These delightful donuts are not only simple to prepare but also rich in protein and low in carbohydrates, making them an ideal choice for your 1200-calorie diet plan Relish a guilt-free dessert that supports your health objectives and helps you stay on course

Ingredients for 1 serving

- 1 scoop vanilla protein powder
- 1/4 cup almond flour
- 1/4 tsp baking powder
- 1/2 tsp cinnamon
- 1 egg white
- 1/4 cup unsweetened almond milk
- 1 tbsp zero-calorie sweetener
- Non-stick cooking spray
- Optional: Cinnamon and sweetener mix for coating

Preparation time and Cooking time

- Preparation time: 10 minutes
- Cooking time: 12 minutes

Directions

1. Preheat your oven to 350°F (175°C) and prepare a donut pan by spraying it with non-stick cooking spray.
2. In a mixing bowl, combine the vanilla protein powder, almond flour, baking powder, and cinnamon.
3. Add the egg white, unsweetened almond milk, and zero-calorie sweetener to the dry ingredients. Mix until well combined into a smooth batter.
4. Transfer the batter into a piping bag or a ziplock bag with a corner cut off to pipe the batter into the donut pan, filling each donut well about 3/4 full.
5. Bake in the preheated oven for 12 minutes, or until a toothpick comes out clean when inserted into a donut.
6. Optional: Once slightly cooled, remove the donuts from the pan and lightly coat them in a mix of cinnamon and sweetener for extra flavor.
7. Let the donuts cool completely on a wire rack before serving.

Nutritional value per serving

- Calories: 180- Carbs: 8g- Fiber: 3g- Sugars: 1g- Protein: 20g- Saturated fat: 0.5g
- Unsaturated fat: 1g

Difficulty rating: ★★☆☆☆

79. PUMPKIN PROTEIN PUDDING

Brief Introduction

Indulge in the creamy delight of Pumpkin Protein Pudding, a perfect dessert to satisfy your sweet cravings without compromising your diet. This recipe combines the seasonal flavor of pumpkin with the nutritional benefits of protein, offering a guilt-free treat that's both delicious and nutritious.

Ingredients for 1 serving

- 1/2 cup pure pumpkin puree
- 1 scoop vanilla protein powder
- 1/2 cup unsweetened almond milk
- 1/4 teaspoon pumpkin pie spice
- 1/4 teaspoon cinnamon
- Stevia or another low-calorie sweetener, to taste

Preparation time and Cooking time

- Preparation time: 5 minutes
- Cooking time: 0 minutes
- Chill time: 1 hour

Directions

1. In a mixing bowl, combine the pumpkin puree and vanilla protein powder. Stir until well mixed.
2. Gradually add the unsweetened almond milk to the mixture, stirring continuously to ensure a smooth consistency.

3. Mix in the pumpkin pie spice, cinnamon, and sweetener, adjusting the sweetener to your taste.
4. Pour the mixture into a serving dish or individual cups.
5. Refrigerate for at least 1 hour to allow the pudding to set and flavors to meld.
6. Serve chilled, optionally garnished with a sprinkle of cinnamon or a dollop of low-fat whipped cream.

Nutritional value per serving

- Calories: 180- Carbs: 12g- Fiber: 3g- Sugars: 4g- Protein: 20g- Saturated fat: 0.5g
- Unsaturated fat: 1g

Difficulty rating: ★★☆☆☆

80. RASPBERRY PROTEIN SORBET

Brief Introduction

Indulge in a refreshing and guilt-free Raspberry Protein Sorbet, perfectly crafted to align with Dr. Nowzaradan's dietary guidelines. This sorbet combines the natural sweetness of raspberries with a protein boost, making it an ideal dessert for those following a high-protein, low-fat, and low-sugar diet. Enjoy the vibrant flavors while staying on track with your health goals.

Ingredients for 1 serving

- 1 cup frozen raspberries
- 1 scoop vanilla protein powder
- 1/4 cup unsweetened almond milk
- 1 tablespoon lemon juice
- Stevia or erythritol to taste

Preparation time and Cooking time

- Preparation time: 5 minutes
- Cooking time: 0 minutes
- Freezing time: 2 hours (if preferred firmer)

Directions

1. Place the frozen raspberries, vanilla protein powder, unsweetened almond milk, and lemon juice in a blender.
2. Blend on high until the mixture is smooth and creamy. Add stevia or erythritol to taste and blend again to incorporate.
3. For a soft-serve texture, serve immediately. For a firmer sorbet, transfer the mixture to a freezer-safe container and freeze for 2 hours.
4. Before serving, let the sorbet sit at room temperature for a few minutes to soften slightly for easier scooping.

Nutritional value per serving

- Calories: 180- Carbs: 18g- Fiber: 8g- Sugars: 8g- Protein: 20g- Saturated fat: 0g
- Unsaturated fat: 1g

Difficulty rating: ★☆☆☆☆

CHAPTER 7: PRACTICAL TIPS

7.1: PORTION CONTROL AND SERVING SIZES

7.1.1: Measure and Control Portions

Measuring and controlling portions is a fundamental aspect of following Dr. Nowzaradan's diet plan effectively. It ensures that you consume the right amount of calories and nutrients without overeating. This process can be simplified by using household items, understanding food labels, and becoming familiar with visual cues for portion sizes.

- **Household Items as Measuring Tools**: You can use common household items as proxies for standard serving sizes. For example, a deck of cards represents a 3-ounce serving of meat, a baseball is about the size of one cup of vegetables, and a computer mouse can approximate a medium-sized piece of fruit.

- **Reading Food Labels**: Always check the serving size on food labels. They provide a clear indication of how much of that food constitutes a single serving and how many calories it contains. This information is crucial for tracking your daily intake and staying within the 1200 calorie limit.

- **Visual Cues for Portion Sizes**: Familiarize yourself with visual cues to estimate serving sizes without measuring tools. For instance, a fist or a cupped hand can represent one cup, a thumb tip is about one teaspoon, and a whole thumb approximates one tablespoon.

- **Weighing Food**: For more accuracy, consider using a kitchen scale to weigh your food, especially for items like meat and fish. This method ensures you're consuming the exact portion sizes recommended in your diet plan.

- **Dividing Your Plate**: A helpful strategy is to divide your plate into sections: half of the plate for vegetables, a quarter for lean proteins, and the remaining quarter for whole grains or starchy vegetables. This visual guide helps in maintaining a balanced diet with controlled portions.

- **Pre-portioned Meals and Snacks**: Preparing meals and snacks in advance in the exact serving sizes can help prevent overeating. Use containers or bags to store these pre-portioned meals and snacks, making it easier to grab the right amount when you're hungry.

- **Mindful Eating**: Pay attention to your hunger and fullness cues. Eating slowly and without distractions allows you to recognize when you're satisfied, reducing the likelihood of overeating.

By incorporating these methods into your daily routine, you can effectively measure and control your portions, which is a key component in achieving and maintaining your weight loss goals on Dr. Nowzaradan's diet plan. Remember, consistency and mindfulness in portion control are as important as the food choices you make.

7.1.2: Serving Sizes Recommendation

Understanding and adhering to recommended serving sizes is crucial for success on Dr. Nowzaradan's diet plan. Proper portion control is not only essential for weight loss but also for maintaining a balanced and nutritious diet. Here are specific serving size recommendations that align with the principles of Dr. Nowzaradan's diet:

- Vegetables: Aim for at least 2 to 3 cups of vegetables per day. This includes leafy greens, cruciferous vegetables like broccoli and cauliflower, and other non-starchy vegetables. A serving size is typically 1 cup for raw leafy vegetables or 1/2 cup for cooked or chopped vegetables.

- Fruits: Limit fruit intake to 1 to 2 servings per day due to their natural sugar content. A serving size is generally 1 medium piece of fruit, such as an apple or banana, or 1/2 cup of chopped fruit.

- Proteins: Include a source of lean protein with each meal, aiming for a total of 4 to 6 ounces per day. A serving size is about 3 ounces for cooked meats, which is roughly the size of a deck of cards.

- Whole Grains: Opt for whole grains and aim for 3 to 4 servings per day, with a serving size being 1/2 cup cooked grains, such as brown rice or quinoa, or 1 slice of whole-grain bread.

- Dairy: Choose low-fat or fat-free dairy products and aim for 2 to 3 servings per day. A serving size is 1 cup of milk or yogurt or 1.5 ounces of cheese.

- Fats: Healthy fats are important but should be consumed in moderation. Aim for 2 to 3 servings per day, with a serving size being 1 teaspoon of oil, 1 tablespoon of salad dressing, or 1/8 of an avocado.

By following these serving size recommendations, individuals can ensure they are consuming a balanced diet that supports weight loss and overall health while adhering to Dr. Nowzaradan's diet principles.

7.2: MANAGING CRAVINGS AND EMOTIONAL EATING

7.2.1: Strategies for Dealing with Cravings

Cravings can be a significant hurdle in maintaining a healthy diet and achieving weight loss goals. They are often a body's way of communicating needs, but not always for the best reasons. Understanding and managing cravings is crucial for sticking to Dr. Nowzaradan's diet plan. Here are strategies to help deal with cravings effectively:

1. **Identify the Trigger**: Recognize what triggers your cravings. Is it emotional, habitual, or due to genuine hunger? Identifying the cause can help you address it directly.

2. **Stay Hydrated**: Sometimes, the body confuses thirst with hunger. Drinking water can help mitigate cravings, especially if they are not based on actual hunger.

3. **Eat Regularly**: Consuming meals and snacks at regular intervals helps stabilize blood sugar levels, reducing the likelihood of experiencing intense cravings.

4. **Opt for Healthy Alternatives**: If you're craving something sweet, opt for a piece of fruit or a serving of Greek Yogurt with Berries. For salty cravings, try a small portion of nuts or seeds.

5. **Practice Mindful Eating**: Pay attention to what you eat and savor each bite. Mindful eating can help satisfy cravings by making meals more fulfilling.

6. **Increase Protein and Fiber Intake**: Foods high in protein and fiber can keep you feeling full longer, which helps curb cravings. Incorporate options like the Egg White Omelette with Spinach and Feta or a Turkey and Veggie Breakfast Wrap into your diet.

7. **Get Active**: Physical activity can help reduce cravings by distracting you and boosting mood.

8. **Ensure Adequate Sleep**: Lack of sleep can increase hunger hormones, leading to cravings. Make sure to get enough rest.

9. **Manage Stress Levels**: Stress can trigger cravings for unhealthy foods. Techniques such as deep breathing, meditation, or yoga can help manage stress.

10. **Allow for an Occasional Treat**: Completely banning your favorite foods can lead to intense cravings. Allowing yourself a small treat occasionally, within the diet's guidelines, can help keep cravings at bay.

By implementing these strategies, you can better manage cravings and stay on track with your diet plan. Remember, consistency is key, and it's okay to have setbacks as long as you continue to strive towards your health goals.

7.2.2: Overcoming Emotional Eating

Emotional eating is a common challenge faced by many individuals on their journey to healthier living. It occurs when food is used as a way to manage or soothe negative emotions, such as stress, anger, fear, boredom, sadness, or loneliness. Instead of eating in response to physical hunger, emotional eating is driven by emotional need. Recognizing and overcoming emotional eating is crucial for adhering to Dr. Nowzaradan's diet plan and achieving long-term weight loss and health goals. Here are practical tips to help overcome emotional eating:

1. **Identify Your Triggers**: Keep a food and mood diary to track when and why you eat. Note what triggers your emotional eating, whether it's a specific event, a time of day, or an emotional state.

2. **Find Alternatives to Eating**: Once you identify your triggers, find healthy alternatives to cope with your emotions. This could include taking a walk, practicing deep-breathing exercises, meditating, calling a friend, or engaging in a hobby.

3. **Eat Mindfully**: Practice mindful eating by paying full attention to the experience of eating. Eat slowly, savor each bite, and eliminate distractions (like TV or reading) to help you recognize fullness and satisfaction cues.

4. **Don't Deprive Yourself**: Restricting yourself too much can lead to cravings and emotional eating. Allow yourself to enjoy occasional treats in moderation within the diet plan. This can help reduce feelings of deprivation.

5. **Build a Support Network**: Share your goals with friends and family who can offer encouragement and support. Consider joining a support group where you can share experiences and strategies with others facing similar challenges.

6. **Develop Stress Management Techniques**: Since stress is a common trigger for emotional eating, finding stress-reduction techniques that work for you is essential. This might include yoga, exercise, journaling, or other relaxation practices.

7. **Ensure Regular, Balanced Meals**: Skipping meals can lead to increased hunger, which may trigger emotional eating. Ensure you eat regular, balanced meals and snacks that align with Dr. Nowzaradan's diet plan to maintain stable blood sugar levels and reduce cravings.

8. **Seek Professional Help**: If emotional eating is deeply rooted or linked to emotional trauma, consider seeking help from a mental health professional. Therapy can provide strategies to cope with emotions in healthier ways.

9. **Practice Self-Compassion**: Be kind to yourself. Understand that setbacks are part of the journey. Acknowledge your progress, learn from experiences, and continue moving forward.

10. **Stay Physically Active**: Regular physical activity can help reduce stress, improve mood, and distract from emotional eating. Find an activity you enjoy and incorporate it into your routine.

By implementing these strategies, you can begin to break the cycle of emotional eating and develop a healthier relationship with food. Remember, overcoming emotional eating is a process that takes time and patience. Stay committed to your health goals, and don't hesitate to seek support when needed.

CHAPTER 8: SPECIAL CONSIDERATIONS AND ADVANCED TIPS

8.1: EATING OUT AND SOCIAL SITUATIONS

8.1.1: Navigating Restaurant Menus

Eating out can be a delightful experience but poses challenges for those following Dr. Nowzaradan's diet plan. The key to success lies in making informed choices that align with the diet's principles of high protein, low carbs, and low fats. Here are strategies to navigate restaurant menus effectively:

1. **Preview the Menu**: Before visiting, review the restaurant's menu online. Look for dishes that fit within the diet's guidelines. This preparation prevents impulsive decisions influenced by hunger or the ambiance.

2. **Ask for Modifications**: Don't hesitate to ask for modifications to your meal. Request dishes to be prepared with less oil or butter, or ask for sauces and dressings on the side. Most restaurants are willing to accommodate such requests.

3. **Choose Protein-Centric Dishes**: Opt for meals that center around lean proteins such as grilled chicken, fish, or tofu. These should take precedence over dishes with high carbohydrate content.

4. **Vegetables as Sides**: Instead of choosing sides like fries or mashed potatoes, ask for steamed vegetables or a salad with a light dressing to keep the meal balanced and within dietary limits.

5. **Beware of Hidden Calories**: Salads can be deceptive; they may contain high-calorie ingredients like croutons, cheese, or creamy dressings. Always inquire about the ingredients and opt for clear dressings like vinaigrettes.

6. **Portion Control**: Restaurant portions can be generous. Consider sharing a dish with a dining companion or immediately boxing half of it to avoid overeating.

7. **Mindful Eating**: Eat slowly and savor each bite. This practice helps in recognizing fullness cues, preventing overindulgence.

8. **Avoid Sugary Beverages**: Choose water, unsweetened tea, or black coffee over sugary drinks or alcohol, which can significantly increase the calorie count of your meal.

By applying these strategies, dining out can still be an enjoyable part of your lifestyle without derailing your progress on Dr. Nowzaradan's diet plan. Making conscious choices ensures that you can navigate any menu while staying committed to your health goals.

8.1.2: Staying Compliant at Social Gatherings

Staying compliant with Dr. Nowzaradan's diet during social gatherings requires planning and strategies to navigate the abundance of tempting foods that may not align with your dietary goals. Here are practical tips to help you maintain your diet and enjoy social events without compromising your health objectives:

- **Choose Wisely**: Focus on foods that are in line with the diet's principles, such as vegetables, lean proteins, and salads without creamy dressings. Avoid fried foods, sugary treats, and high-carb options.

- **Eat Before You Go**: Having a small, healthy meal or snack before attending a social event can reduce your hunger and the temptation to indulge in less healthy options.

- **Bring Your Own Dish**: If it's a potluck, bring a dish that fits your diet plan. This ensures you'll have at least one item you can enjoy without guilt.

- **Stay Hydrated**: Drink plenty of water throughout the event. Sometimes thirst is mistaken for hunger. Water can also help you feel full and avoid unnecessary snacking.

- **Practice Portion Control**: If you choose to try foods outside your usual diet, do so in small amounts. This can help satisfy your craving without significantly impacting your dietary goals.

- **Focus on Socializing**: Remember, the primary purpose of social gatherings is to interact with others. Focus on conversations rather than the food.

- **Politely Decline**: It's okay to say no to food offers that don't meet your dietary needs. Most hosts will understand your commitment to maintaining a healthy lifestyle.

By applying these strategies, you can navigate social gatherings confidently, knowing you're making choices that support your health and dietary goals.

8.2: ADAPTING THE DIET FOR SPECIAL NEEDS

8.2.1: Modifying Recipes for Dietary Restrictions

Adapting recipes to meet dietary restrictions is essential for ensuring that everyone can enjoy delicious, nutritious meals that align with their health needs and preferences. Whether due to allergies, intolerances, religious practices, or personal choices, modifying recipes allows for inclusivity and variety in any diet plan. This section provides guidance on how to adjust the recipes within this book to accommodate common dietary restrictions, ensuring that the meals remain within the principles of Dr. Nowzaradan's diet plan.

Dairy-Free Modifications
- Substitute dairy products like milk, yogurt, and cheese with plant-based alternatives such as almond milk, coconut yogurt, and nutritional yeast.
- For the "Greek Yogurt Parfait with Berries," use coconut yogurt instead of Greek yogurt.

Gluten-Free Adjustments
- Replace any wheat-based products with gluten-free alternatives. For instance, use gluten-free wraps for the "Turkey and Veggie Breakfast Wrap."
- Ensure that all packaged ingredients are certified gluten-free to avoid cross-contamination.

Vegetarian and Vegan Variations
- Replace animal proteins with plant-based proteins. Tofu, tempeh, and legumes are excellent choices.
- For the "Grilled Lemon Herb Chicken," use marinated tofu or tempeh as a substitute for chicken.
- Use vegan cheese and dairy substitutes where necessary.

Low-Sodium Solutions
- Reduce or eliminate added salt. Use herbs and spices to enhance flavor without increasing sodium content.
- For recipes like the "Spicy Tuna and Avocado Wrap," opt for low-sodium canned tuna and limit the addition of salt.

Nut-Free Options
- Omit nuts from recipes or use seeds as a safe alternative for those with nut allergies.
- In the "Overnight Chia Pudding with Almonds," replace almonds with sunflower seeds or simply omit them.

Sugar-Free Substitutes
- For recipes requiring sweeteners, use stevia, erythritol, or monk fruit sweetener as sugar-free alternatives.
- Modify the "High-Protein Chocolate Mousse" by using a sugar-free chocolate and sweetener instead of regular chocolate and sugar.

Adjusting for Paleo and Keto Diets
- Focus on eliminating grains, legumes, and high-carb fruits from recipes for those following Paleo or Keto diets.
- Adapt the "Quinoa Breakfast Bowl with Veggies" by replacing quinoa with cauliflower rice.

Preparation and Cooking Adjustments

- Preparation time and cooking time may vary slightly with substitutions. Always monitor cooking progress to ensure optimal results.
- Difficulty rating may increase slightly with modifications due to the need for additional preparation of substitute ingredients.

Nutritional Values
- Nutritional values will vary based on substitutions. Use a nutritional calculator to estimate the values of the modified recipe to ensure it aligns with dietary goals.
- Ensure that the modified recipes still align with the caloric and macronutrient guidelines of Dr. Nowzaradan's diet plan.

By carefully selecting alternative ingredients, it's possible to modify recipes to cater to a wide range of dietary restrictions while still adhering to the principles of a healthy, balanced diet.

120-DAY MEAL PLAN

Day 1
- **Breakfast**: Greek Yogurt Parfait with Berries (230 Calories)
- **Lunch**: Grilled Chicken and Veggie Wrap (320 Calories)
- **Snack**: Protein-Packed Lemon Cheesecake Bites (180 Calories)
- **Dinner**: Grilled Lemon Herb Chicken with Zucchini Noodles (250 Calories)
- **Dessert**: Vanilla Protein Pudding with Cinnamon (200 Calories)
- **Total Calories**: 1180

Day 2
- **Breakfast**: Scrambled Tofu with Vegetables (200 Calories)
- **Lunch**: Spicy Tuna and Avocado Wrap (330 Calories)
- **Snack**: Greek Yogurt and Berry Parfait (160 Calories)
- **Dinner**: Lemon Herb Quinoa Salad (330 Calories)
- **Dessert**: High-Protein Chocolate Mousse (180 Calories)
- **Total Calories**: 1200

Day 3
- **Breakfast**: High-Protein Apple Cinnamon Muffins (160 Calories)
- **Lunch**: Turkey and Hummus Roll-Ups (320 Calories)
- **Snack**: Peanut Butter Protein Balls (180 Calories)
- **Dinner**: Spicy Chicken and Cucumber Salad (300 Calories)
- **Dessert**: Low-Fat Ricotta and Lemon Tart (200 Calories)
- **Total Calories**: 1160

Day 4
- **Breakfast**: Greek Yogurt with Cucumber and Herbs (120 Calories)
- **Lunch**: Chicken and Quinoa Salad (320 Calories)
- **Snack**: Protein-Packed Peanut Butter Cookies (180 Calories)
- **Dinner**: Grilled Chicken and Veggie Skewers (300 Calories)
- **Dessert**: High-Protein Chocolate Lava Cake (200 Calories)
- **Total Calories**: 1120

Day 5
- **Breakfast**: Scrambled Tofu with Vegetables (200 Calories)
- **Lunch**: Shrimp and Avocado Salad (300 Calories)
- **Snack**: Protein-Packed Lemon Cheesecake Bites (180 Calories)
- **Dinner**: Grilled Lemon Herb Shrimp (300 Calories)
- **Dessert**: Vanilla Protein Pudding (180 Calories)
- **Total Calories**: 1160

Day 6
- **Breakfast**: High-Protein Apple Cinnamon Muffins (160 Calories)
- **Lunch**: Grilled Chicken Caesar Salad (300 Calories)
- **Snack**: Strawberry Almond Cottage Cheese Bliss (165 Calories)
- **Dinner**: Grilled Chicken and Veggie Skewers (300 Calories)
- **Dessert**: Greek Yogurt Cheesecake with Fresh Berries (200 Calories)
- **Total Calories**: 1125

Day 7
- **Breakfast**: Egg White Omelette with Spinach and Feta (180 Calories)
- **Lunch**: Tuna Salad Lettuce Wraps (200 Calories)
- **Snack**: Almond Flour Chocolate Brownies (200 Calories)
- **Dinner**: Grilled Shrimp with Cauliflower Rice (270 Calories)
- **Dessert**: Greek Yogurt Cheesecake with Fresh Berries (200 Calories)
- **Total Calories**: 1150

Day 8
- **Breakfast**: Greek Yogurt Parfait with Berries (230 Calories)
- **Lunch**: Grilled Chicken and Veggie Skewers (320 Calories)
- **Snack**: Protein-Packed Lemon Cheesecake Bites (180 Calories)
- **Dinner**: Grilled Tofu with Steamed Broccoli (230 Calories)
- **Dessert**: Protein-Packed Chocolate Chip Cookies (200 Calories)
- **Total Calories**: 1160

Day 9
- **Breakfast**: Egg White and Veggie Breakfast Sandwich (250 Calories)
- **Lunch**: Shrimp and Cauliflower Rice Stir-Fry (250 Calories)
- **Snack**: Cottage Cheese and Pineapple Delight (150 Calories)
- **Dinner**: Grilled Salmon with Asparagus (290 Calories)
- **Dessert**: Greek Yogurt Cheesecake with Fresh Berries (200 Calories)
- **Total Calories**: 1140

Day 10
- **Breakfast**: Protein-Packed Smoothie (230 Calories)
- **Lunch**: Turkey and Hummus Roll-Ups (320 Calories)
- **Snack**: High-Protein Apple Cinnamon Muffins (180 Calories)
- **Dinner**: Grilled Chicken and Zucchini Noodles (250 Calories)
- **Dessert**: Vanilla Protein Pudding with Cinnamon (200 Calories)
- **Total Calories**: 1180

Day 11
- **Breakfast**: Smoked Salmon and Avocado Toast (240 Calories)
- **Lunch**: Chicken and Quinoa Salad (320 Calories)
- **Snack**: Greek Yogurt and Berry Parfait (170 Calories)
- **Dinner**: Grilled Shrimp and Veggie Skewers (260 Calories)
- **Dessert**: Low-Fat Ricotta and Lemon Tart (200 Calories)
- **Total Calories**: 1190

Day 12
- **Breakfast**: Overnight Chia Pudding with Almonds (250 Calories)
- **Lunch**: Turkey and Spinach Roll-Ups (320 Calories)
- **Snack**: Greek Yogurt with Cucumber and Herbs (120 Calories)
- **Dinner**: Turkey Meatballs with Spaghetti Squash (290 Calories)
- **Dessert**: Almond Flour Chocolate Brownies (200 Calories)
- **Total Calories**: 1180

Day 13
- **Breakfast**: Turkey and Veggie Breakfast Wrap (250 Calories)
- **Lunch**: Grilled Chicken and Veggie Skewers (300 Calories)
- **Snack**: Cottage Cheese and Berry Bowl (150 Calories)
- **Dinner**: Baked Cod with Green Beans (250 Calories)
- **Dessert**: High-Protein Chocolate Lava Cake (200 Calories)
- **Total Calories**: 1150

Day 14
- **Breakfast**: Low-Fat Greek Yogurt with Fresh Fruit (230 Calories)
- **Lunch**: Chicken and Black Bean Salad (345 Calories)
- **Snack**: Protein-Packed Peanut Butter Cookies (180 Calories)
- **Dinner**: Grilled Salmon with Brussels Sprouts (280 Calories)
- **Dessert**: Protein-Packed Chocolate Chip Cookies (200 Calories)
- **Total Calories**: 1190

Day 15
- **Breakfast**: Greek Yogurt Parfait with Berries (230 Calories)
- **Lunch**: Grilled Chicken and Veggie Wrap (320 Calories)
- **Snack**: Protein-Packed Lemon Cheesecake Bites (180 Calories)
- **Dinner**: Grilled Lemon Herb Chicken with Zucchini Noodles (250 Calories)
- **Dessert**: Greek Yogurt Cheesecake with Fresh Berries (200 Calories)
- **Total Calories**: 1180

Day 16
- **Breakfast**: Egg White and Veggie Breakfast Sandwich (250 Calories)
- **Lunch**: Tuna Salad Lettuce Wraps (200 Calories)
- **Snack**: High-Protein Chocolate Mousse (180 Calories)
- **Dinner**: Baked Cod with Asparagus (250 Calories)
- **Dessert**: Low-Fat Ricotta and Lemon Tart (200 Calories)
- **Total Calories**: 1180

Day 17
- **Breakfast**: Protein-Packed Smoothie (230 Calories)
- **Lunch**: Turkey and Hummus Roll-Ups (320 Calories)
- **Snack**: Spicy Roasted Chickpeas (150 Calories)
- **Dinner**: Turkey Meatballs with Spaghetti Squash (290 Calories)
- **Dessert**: Protein-Packed Chocolate Chip Cookies (200 Calories)
- **Total Calories**: 1190

Day 18
- **Breakfast**: Smoked Salmon and Avocado Toast (240 Calories)
- **Lunch**: Chicken and Quinoa Salad (320 Calories)
- **Snack**: Cottage Cheese and Pineapple Delight (160 Calories)
- **Dinner**: Grilled Lemon Herb Chicken (250 Calories)
- **Dessert**: Almond Flour Chocolate Brownies (200 Calories)
- **Total Calories**: 1170

Day 19
- **Breakfast**: Overnight Chia Pudding with Almonds (250 Calories)
- **Lunch**: Shrimp and Avocado Salad (300 Calories)
- **Snack**: Tofu Veggie Bites (140 Calories)
- **Dinner**: Chicken and Zucchini Noodles (230 Calories)
- **Dessert**: Vanilla Protein Pudding with Cinnamon (200 Calories)
- **Total Calories**: 1120

Day 20
- **Breakfast**: Low-Fat Greek Yogurt with Fresh Fruit (230 Calories)
- **Lunch**: Chicken and Black Bean Salad (345 Calories)
- **Snack**: Protein-Packed Chocolate Chip Cookies (200 Calories)
- **Dinner**: Grilled Salmon with Asparagus (290 Calories)
- **Dessert**: Vanilla Protein Pudding with Cinnamon (200 Calories)
- **Total Calories**: 1200

Day 21
- **Breakfast**: Low-Fat Greek Yogurt with Fresh Fruit (230 Calories)
- **Lunch**: Chicken and Black Bean Salad (345 Calories)
- **Snack**: Greek Yogurt and Cucumber Dip with Veggies (140 Calories)
- **Dinner**: Grilled Salmon with Green Beans (290 Calories)
- **Dessert**: High-Protein Chocolate Lava Cake (200 Calories)
- **Total Calories**: 1205

Day 22
- **Breakfast**: Greek Yogurt Parfait with Berries (230 Calories)
- **Lunch**: Grilled Chicken and Veggie Wrap (320 Calories)
- **Snack**: Protein-Packed Lemon Cheesecake Bites (180 Calories)
- **Dinner**: Grilled Lemon Herb Chicken with Zucchini Noodles (250 Calories)
- **Dessert**: Vanilla Protein Pudding with Cinnamon (200 Calories)
- **Total Calories**: 1180

Day 23

- **Breakfast**: Egg White Omelette with Spinach and Feta (180 Calories)
- **Lunch**: Tuna Salad Lettuce Wraps (200 Calories)
- **Snack**: Greek Yogurt with Cucumber and Herbs (120 Calories)
- **Dinner**: Grilled Shrimp with Cauliflower Rice (270 Calories)
- **Dessert**: High-Protein Chocolate Lava Cake (200 Calories)
- **Total Calories**: 1170

Day 24

- **Breakfast**: Protein-Packed Smoothie with Almond Milk and Berries (230 Calories)
- **Lunch**: Turkey and Hummus Roll-Ups (320 Calories)
- **Snack**: Cottage Cheese and Pineapple Delight (150 Calories)
- **Dinner**: Grilled Chicken with Zucchini Noodles (250 Calories)
- **Dessert**: Greek Yogurt Cheesecake with Fresh Berries (200 Calories)
- **Total Calories**: 1150

Day 25

- **Breakfast**: Low-Fat Greek Yogurt with Fresh Fruit (230 Calories)
- **Lunch**: Chicken and Black Bean Salad (345 Calories)
- **Snack**: Cottage Cheese and Berry Bowl (150 Calories)
- **Dinner**: Grilled Salmon with Asparagus (290 Calories)
- **Dessert**: High-Protein Chocolate Lava Cake (200 Calories)
- **Total Calories**: 1195

Day 26

- **Breakfast**: Overnight Chia Pudding with Almonds (250 Calories)
- **Lunch**: Shrimp and Avocado Salad (300 Calories)
- **Snack**: High-Protein Chocolate Mousse (170 Calories)
- **Dinner**: Turkey Meatballs with Spaghetti Squash (290 Calories)
- **Dessert**: Greek Yogurt Cheesecake with Fresh Berries (200 Calories)
- **Total Calories**: 1210

Day 27

- **Breakfast**: Turkey and Veggie Breakfast Wrap (250 Calories)
- **Lunch**: Turkey and Spinach Roll-Ups (320 Calories)
- **Snack**: Greek Yogurt with Cucumber and Herbs (120 Calories)
- **Dinner**: Grilled Shrimp with Veggie Stir-Fry (250 Calories)
- **Dessert**: Low-Fat Ricotta and Lemon Tart (200 Calories)
- **Total Calories**: 1140

Day 28

- **Breakfast**: Low-Fat Greek Yogurt with Fresh Fruit (230 Calories)
- **Lunch**: Chicken and Black Bean Salad (345 Calories)
- **Snack**: Almond Flour Chocolate Brownies (200 Calories)
- **Dinner**: Grilled Salmon with Asparagus (290 Calories)
- **Dessert**: Vanilla Protein Pudding with Cinnamon (200 Calories)
- **Total Calories**: 1175

Day 29

- **Breakfast**: Greek Yogurt Parfait with Berries (230 Calories)
- **Lunch**: Grilled Chicken and Veggie Wrap (320 Calories)
- **Snack**: Protein-Packed Peanut Butter Cookies (180 Calories)
- **Dinner**: Grilled Lemon Herb Chicken with Steamed Broccoli (250 Calories)
- **Dessert**: High-Protein Chocolate Lava Cake (200 Calories)
- **Total Calories**: 1180

Day 30

- **Breakfast**: Egg White Omelette with Spinach and Feta (180 Calories)
- **Lunch**: Tuna Salad Lettuce Wraps (200 Calories)
- **Snack**: Almond Butter and Banana Rice Cakes (245 Calories)
- **Dinner**: Grilled Shrimp with Cauliflower Rice (270 Calories)
- **Dessert**: Low-Fat Ricotta and Lemon Tart (200 Calories)
- **Total Calories**: 1195

Day 31
- **Breakfast**: Protein-Packed Smoothie with Almond Milk and Berries (230 Calories)
- **Lunch**: Turkey and Hummus Roll-Ups (320 Calories)
- **Snack**: Greek Yogurt with Cucumber and Herbs (120 Calories)
- **Dinner**: Grilled Chicken and Zucchini Noodles (250 Calories)
- **Dessert**: Vanilla Protein Pudding with Cinnamon (200 Calories)
- **Total Calories**: 1120

Day 32
- **Breakfast**: Smoked Salmon and Avocado Toast (240 Calories)
- **Lunch**: Chicken and Quinoa Salad (320 Calories)
- **Snack**: Cottage Cheese and Berry Smoothie (200 Calories)
- **Dinner**: Grilled Salmon with Steamed Green Beans (290 Calories)
- **Dessert**: Protein-Packed Chocolate Chip Cookies (200 Calories)
- **Total Calories**: 1250

Day 33
- **Breakfast**: Overnight Chia Pudding with Almonds (250 Calories)
- **Lunch**: Shrimp and Avocado Salad (300 Calories)
- **Snack**: Peanut Butter Protein Balls (180 Calories)
- **Dinner**: Turkey Meatballs with Spaghetti Squash (290 Calories)
- **Dessert**: Greek Yogurt Cheesecake with Fresh Berries (200 Calories)
- **Total Calories**: 1220

Day 34
- **Breakfast**: Turkey and Veggie Breakfast Wrap (250 Calories)
- **Lunch**: Turkey and Spinach Roll-Ups (320 Calories)
- **Snack**: Protein-Packed Lemon Cheesecake Bites (180 Calories)
- **Dinner**: Grilled Shrimp with Veggie Stir-Fry (250 Calories)
- **Dessert**: High-Protein Chocolate Lava Cake (200 Calories)
- **Total Calories**: 1200

Day 35
- **Breakfast**: Low-Fat Greek Yogurt with Fresh Fruit (230 Calories)
- **Lunch**: Chicken and Black Bean Salad (345 Calories)
- **Snack**: Cottage Cheese and Pineapple Delight (160 Calories)
- **Dinner**: Grilled Salmon with Asparagus (290 Calories)
- **Dessert**: Almond Flour Chocolate Brownies (200 Calories)
- **Total Calories**: 1225

Day 36
- **Breakfast**: High-Protein Banana Pancakes (240 Calories)
- **Lunch**: Grilled Chicken and Veggie Wrap (320 Calories)
- **Snack**: Protein-Packed Peanut Butter Cookies (180 Calories)
- **Dinner**: Grilled Lemon Herb Chicken with Zucchini Noodles (250 Calories)
- **Dessert**: Greek Yogurt Cheesecake with Fresh Berries (200 Calories)
- **Total Calories**: 1190

Day 37
- **Breakfast**: Scrambled Tofu with Vegetables (200 Calories)
- **Lunch**: Tuna Salad Lettuce Wraps (200 Calories)
- **Snack**: Protein-Packed Lemon Cheesecake Bites (180 Calories)
- **Dinner**: Grilled Shrimp with Cauliflower Rice (270 Calories)
- **Dessert**: Low-Fat Ricotta and Lemon Tart (200 Calories)
- **Total Calories**: 1150

Day 38
- **Breakfast**: Greek Yogurt Parfait with Berries (230 Calories)
- **Lunch**: Turkey and Hummus Roll-Ups (320 Calories)
- **Snack**: Cottage Cheese and Pineapple Delight (150 Calories)
- **Dinner**: Grilled Salmon with Steamed Broccoli (290 Calories)
- **Dessert**: Vanilla Protein Pudding with Cinnamon (200 Calories)
- **Total Calories**: 1190

Day 39
- **Breakfast**: Smoked Salmon and Avocado Toast (240 Calories)
- **Lunch**: Chicken and Quinoa Salad (320 Calories)
- **Snack**: Greek Yogurt with Cucumber and Herbs (120 Calories)
- **Dinner**: Turkey Meatballs with Spaghetti Squash (290 Calories)
- **Dessert**: High-Protein Chocolate Lava Cake (200 Calories)
- **Total Calories**: 1170

Day 40
- **Breakfast**: Protein-Packed Smoothie (230 Calories)
- **Lunch**: Grilled Chicken Caesar Salad (300 Calories)
- **Snack**: Greek Yogurt and Berry Parfait (160 Calories)
- **Dinner**: Baked Cod with Asparagus (250 Calories)
- **Dessert**: Greek Yogurt Cheesecake with Fresh Berries (200 Calories)
- **Total Calories**: 1140

Day 41
- **Breakfast**: Egg White and Veggie Breakfast Sandwich (250 Calories)
- **Lunch**: Shrimp and Avocado Salad (300 Calories)
- **Snack**: High-Protein Chocolate Mousse (160 Calories)
- **Dinner**: Grilled Chicken with Steamed Green Beans (280 Calories)
- **Dessert**: Protein-Packed Chocolate Chip Cookies (200 Calories)
- **Total Calories**: 1190

Day 42
- **Breakfast**: Low-Fat Greek Yogurt with Fresh Fruit (230 Calories)
- **Lunch**: Chicken and Black Bean Salad (345 Calories)
- **Snack**: Peanut Butter Protein Balls (180 Calories)
- **Dinner**: Grilled Lemon Herb Shrimp with Veggies (290 Calories)
- **Dessert**: Almond Flour Chocolate Brownies (200 Calories)
- **Total Calories**: 1245

Day 43
- **Breakfast**: Greek Yogurt Parfait with Berries (230 Calories)
- **Lunch**: Grilled Chicken and Veggie Wrap (320 Calories)
- **Snack**: Protein-Packed Chocolate Chip Cookies (200 Calories)
- **Dinner**: Grilled Lemon Herb Chicken with Zucchini Noodles (250 Calories)
- **Dessert**: Vanilla Protein Pudding with Cinnamon (200 Calories)
- **Total Calories**: 1200

Day 44
- **Breakfast**: Egg White Omelette with Spinach and Feta (200 Calories)
- **Lunch**: Shrimp and Avocado Salad (300 Calories)
- **Snack**: High-Protein Apple Cinnamon Muffins (160 Calories)
- **Dinner**: Grilled Lemon Herb Shrimp with Zucchini Noodles (250 Calories)
- **Dessert**: High-Protein Chocolate Lava Cake (200 Calories)
- **Total Calories**: 1160

Day 45
- **Breakfast**: Protein-Packed Smoothie with Almond Milk and Berries (230 Calories)
- **Lunch**: Turkey and Hummus Roll-Ups (320 Calories)
- **Snack**: Cottage Cheese and Pineapple Delight (150 Calories)
- **Dinner**: Grilled Salmon with Steamed Broccoli (290 Calories)
- **Dessert**: Vanilla Protein Pudding with Cinnamon (200 Calories)
- **Total Calories**: 1190

Day 46
- **Breakfast**: Smoked Salmon and Avocado Toast (240 Calories)
- **Lunch**: Chicken and Quinoa Salad (320 Calories)
- **Snack**: Greek Yogurt with Cucumber and Herbs (120 Calories)
- **Dinner**: Turkey Meatballs with Spaghetti Squash (290 Calories)
- **Dessert**: Low-Fat Ricotta and Lemon Tart (200 Calories)
- **Total Calories**: 1170

Day 47
- **Breakfast**: Overnight Chia Pudding with Almonds (250 Calories)
- **Lunch**: Grilled Chicken Caesar Salad (300 Calories)
- **Snack**: Protein-Packed Lemon Cheesecake Bites (180 Calories)
- **Dinner**: Grilled Shrimp with Veggies (250 Calories)
- **Dessert**: Protein-Packed Chocolate Chip Cookies (200 Calories)
- **Total Calories**: 1180

Day 48
- **Breakfast**: Turkey and Veggie Breakfast Wrap (250 Calories)
- **Lunch**: Turkey and Spinach Roll-Ups (320 Calories)
- **Snack**: Peanut Butter Protein Balls (180 Calories)
- **Dinner**: Grilled Chicken with Steamed Green Beans (280 Calories)
- **Dessert**: Greek Yogurt Cheesecake with Fresh Berries (200 Calories)
- **Total Calories**: 1230

Day 49
- **Breakfast**: Low-Fat Greek Yogurt with Fresh Fruit (230 Calories)
- **Lunch**: Chicken and Black Bean Salad (345 Calories)
- **Snack**: Almond Flour Chocolate Brownies (200 Calories)
- **Dinner**: Grilled Lemon Herb Shrimp with Veggies (290 Calories)
- **Dessert**: Vanilla Protein Pudding with Cinnamon (200 Calories)
- **Total Calories**: 1185

Day 50
- **Breakfast**: Greek Yogurt Parfait with Berries (230 Calories)
- **Lunch**: Grilled Chicken and Veggie Wrap (320 Calories)
- **Snack**: Protein-Packed Lemon Cheesecake Bites (180 Calories)
- **Dinner**: Grilled Lemon Herb Chicken with Zucchini Noodles (250 Calories)
- **Dessert**: Greek Yogurt Cheesecake with Fresh Berries (200 Calories)
- **Total Calories**: 1180

Day 51
- **Breakfast**: Egg White Omelette with Spinach and Feta (180 Calories)
- **Lunch**: Tuna Salad Lettuce Wraps (200 Calories)
- **Snack**: Cottage Cheese with Pineapple (150 Calories)
- **Dinner**: Grilled Shrimp with Cauliflower Rice (270 Calories)
- **Dessert**: Almond Flour Chocolate Brownies (200 Calories)
- **Total Calories**: 1200

Day 52
- **Breakfast**: Protein-Packed Smoothie with Almond Milk and Berries (230 Calories)
- **Lunch**: Turkey and Hummus Roll-Ups (320 Calories)
- **Snack**: Cucumber Slices with Hummus (100 Calories)
- **Dinner**: Grilled Chicken with Zucchini Noodles (250 Calories)
- **Dessert**: Vanilla Protein Pudding with Cinnamon (200 Calories)
- **Total Calories**: 1200

Day 53
- **Breakfast**: Smoked Salmon and Avocado Toast (240 Calories)
- **Lunch**: Chicken and Quinoa Salad (320 Calories)
- **Snack**: Low-Fat Ricotta and Lemon Tart (200 Calories)
- **Dinner**: Grilled Salmon with Steamed Broccoli (290 Calories)
- **Dessert**: Protein-Packed Chocolate Chip Cookies (200 Calories)
- **Total Calories**: 1250

Day 54
- **Breakfast**: Overnight Chia Pudding with Almonds (250 Calories)
- **Lunch**: Shrimp and Avocado Salad (300 Calories)
- **Snack**: Greek Yogurt with Cucumber and Herbs (150 Calories)
- **Dinner**: Turkey Meatballs with Spaghetti Squash (290 Calories)
- **Dessert**: High-Protein Chocolate Lava Cake (200 Calories)
- **Total Calories**: 1240

Day 55
- **Breakfast**: Turkey and Veggie Breakfast Wrap (250 Calories)
- **Lunch**: Turkey and Spinach Roll-Ups (320 Calories)
- **Snack**: Low-Fat Greek Yogurt with Berries (120 Calories)
- **Dinner**: Grilled Shrimp with Veggie Stir-Fry (250 Calories)
- **Dessert**: Almond Flour Chocolate Brownies (200 Calories)
- **Total Calories**: 1140

Day 56
- **Breakfast**: Low-Fat Greek Yogurt with Fresh Fruit (230 Calories)
- **Lunch**: Chicken and Black Bean Salad (345 Calories)
- **Snack**: Protein-Packed Chocolate Chip Cookies (150 Calories)
- **Dinner**: Grilled Salmon with Asparagus (290 Calories)
- **Dessert**: Vanilla Protein Pudding with Cinnamon (200 Calories)
- **Total Calories**: 1215

Day 57
- **Breakfast**: Greek Yogurt Parfait with Berries (230 Calories)
- **Lunch**: Grilled Chicken and Veggie Wrap (320 Calories)
- **Snack**: Protein-Packed Lemon Cheesecake Bites (180 Calories)
- **Dinner**: Grilled Lemon Herb Chicken with Steamed Broccoli (250 Calories)
- **Dessert**: Greek Yogurt Cheesecake with Fresh Berries (200 Calories)
- **Total Calories**: 1180

Day 58
- **Breakfast**: Egg White Omelette with Spinach and Feta (200 Calories)
- **Lunch**: Tuna Salad Lettuce Wraps (200 Calories)
- **Snack**: High-Protein Apple Cinnamon Muffins (160 Calories)
- **Dinner**: Grilled Lemon Herb Shrimp with Zucchini Noodles (250 Calories)
- **Dessert**: High-Protein Chocolate Lava Cake (200 Calories)
- **Total Calories**: 1160

Day 59
- **Breakfast**: Protein-Packed Smoothie with Almond Milk and Berries (230 Calories)
- **Lunch**: Turkey and Hummus Roll-Ups (320 Calories)
- **Snack**: Cottage Cheese and Pineapple Delight (150 Calories)
- **Dinner**: Grilled Salmon with Steamed Broccoli (290 Calories)
- **Dessert**: Vanilla Protein Pudding with Cinnamon (200 Calories)
- **Total Calories**: 1190

Day 60
- **Breakfast**: Smoked Salmon and Avocado Toast (240 Calories)
- **Lunch**: Chicken and Quinoa Salad (320 Calories)
- **Snack**: Greek Yogurt with Cucumber and Herbs (120 Calories)
- **Dinner**: Turkey Meatballs with Spaghetti Squash (290 Calories)
- **Dessert**: Low-Fat Ricotta and Lemon Tart (200 Calories)
- **Total Calories**: 1170

Day 61
- **Breakfast**: Overnight Chia Pudding with Almonds (250 Calories)
- **Lunch**: Grilled Chicken Caesar Salad (300 Calories)
- **Snack**: Protein-Packed Lemon Cheesecake Bites (180 Calories)
- **Dinner**: Grilled Shrimp with Veggies (250 Calories)
- **Dessert**: Protein-Packed Chocolate Chip Cookies (200 Calories)
- **Total Calories**: 1180

Day 62
- **Breakfast**: Turkey and Veggie Breakfast Wrap (250 Calories)
- **Lunch**: Turkey and Spinach Roll-Ups (320 Calories)
- **Snack**: Peanut Butter Protein Balls (180 Calories)
- **Dinner**: Grilled Chicken with Steamed Green Beans (280 Calories)
- **Dessert**: Greek Yogurt Cheesecake with Fresh Berries (200 Calories)
- **Total Calories**: 1190

Day 63
- **Breakfast**: Low-Fat Greek Yogurt with Fresh Fruit (230 Calories)
- **Lunch**: Chicken and Black Bean Salad (345 Calories)
- **Snack**: Almond Flour Chocolate Brownies (200 Calories)
- **Dinner**: Grilled Lemon Herb Shrimp with Veggies (290 Calories)
- **Dessert**: Vanilla Protein Pudding with Cinnamon (200 Calories)
- **Total Calories**: 1185

Day 64
- **Breakfast**: Greek Yogurt Parfait with Berries (230 Calories)
- **Lunch**: Grilled Chicken and Veggie Wrap (320 Calories)
- **Snack**: Protein-Packed Peanut Butter Cookies (180 Calories)
- **Dinner**: Grilled Lemon Herb Chicken with Steamed Broccoli (250 Calories)
- **Dessert**: Vanilla Protein Pudding with Cinnamon (200 Calories)
- **Total Calories**: 1180

Day 65
- **Breakfast**: Scrambled Egg Whites with Spinach and Feta (200 Calories)
- **Lunch**: Turkey and Hummus Roll-Ups (320 Calories)
- **Snack**: Cottage Cheese and Pineapple Delight (150 Calories)
- **Dinner**: Grilled Shrimp with Cauliflower Rice (270 Calories)
- **Dessert**: Greek Yogurt Cheesecake with Fresh Berries (200 Calories)
- **Total Calories**: 1140

Day 66
- **Breakfast**: Protein-Packed Smoothie (230 Calories)
- **Lunch**: Grilled Salmon with Steamed Broccoli (320 Calories)
- **Snack**: High-Protein Apple Cinnamon Muffins (160 Calories)
- **Dinner**: Grilled Chicken with Zucchini Noodles (250 Calories)
- **Dessert**: Low-Fat Ricotta and Lemon Tart (200 Calories)
- **Total Calories**: 1160

Day 67
- **Breakfast**: Smoked Salmon and Avocado Toast (240 Calories)
- **Lunch**: Chicken and Quinoa Salad (320 Calories)
- **Snack**: Greek Yogurt with Cucumber and Herbs (120 Calories)
- **Dinner**: Grilled Lemon Herb Shrimp with Zucchini Noodles (250 Calories)
- **Dessert**: High-Protein Chocolate Lava Cake (200 Calories)
- **Total Calories**: 1130

Day 68
- **Breakfast**: Overnight Chia Pudding with Almonds (250 Calories)
- **Lunch**: Grilled Chicken Caesar Salad (300 Calories)
- **Snack**: Protein-Packed Lemon Cheesecake Bites (180 Calories)
- **Dinner**: Grilled Shrimp with Veggie Stir-Fry (250 Calories)
- **Dessert**: Almond Flour Chocolate Brownies (200 Calories)
- **Total Calories**: 1180

Day 69
- **Breakfast**: Turkey and Veggie Breakfast Wrap (250 Calories)
- **Lunch**: Turkey and Spinach Roll-Ups (320 Calories)
- **Snack**: Protein-Packed Peanut Butter Cookies (180 Calories)
- **Dinner**: Grilled Chicken with Steamed Green Beans (280 Calories)
- **Dessert**: Greek Yogurt Cheesecake with Fresh Berries (200 Calories)
- **Total Calories**: 1190

Day 70
- **Breakfast**: Low-Fat Greek Yogurt with Fresh Fruit (230 Calories)
- **Lunch**: Chicken and Black Bean Salad (345 Calories)
- **Snack**: Almond Flour Chocolate Brownies (200 Calories)
- **Dinner**: Grilled Lemon Herb Shrimp with Veggies (290 Calories)
- **Dessert**: Vanilla Protein Pudding with Cinnamon (200 Calories)
- **Total Calories**: 1165

Day 71
- **Breakfast**: Greek Yogurt with Cucumber and Herbs (120 Calories)
- **Lunch**: Turkey and Spinach Pinwheels (320 Calories)
- **Snack**: Cottage Cheese and Berry Bowl (200 Calories)
- **Dinner**: Grilled Lemon Herb Chicken (300 Calories)
- **Dessert**: Low-Fat Ricotta and Berry Toast (200 Calories)
- **Total Calories**: 1140

Day 72
- **Breakfast**: Egg White Omelette with Spinach and Feta (180 Calories)
- **Lunch**: Grilled Chicken and Veggie Wrap (300 Calories)
- **Snack**: Protein-Packed Smoothie with Almond Milk and Berries (230 Calories)
- **Dinner**: Turkey Meatballs with Spaghetti Squash (280 Calories)
- **Dessert**: Greek Yogurt Cheesecake with Fresh Berries (200 Calories)
- **Total Calories**: 1190

Day 73
- **Breakfast**: Cottage Cheese and Berry Bowl (200 Calories)
- **Lunch**: Chicken and Quinoa Salad (330 Calories)
- **Snack**: Greek Yogurt with Stevia and Walnuts (245 Calories)
- **Dinner**: Grilled Shrimp and Veggie Skewers (300 Calories)
- **Dessert**: High-Protein Chocolate Lava Cake (125 Calories)
- **Total Calories**: 1200

Day 74
- **Breakfast**: Protein-Packed Smoothie with Almond Milk and Berries (230 Calories)
- **Lunch**: Turkey and Cucumber Roll-Ups (150 Calories)
- **Snack**: Low-Fat Greek Yogurt with Fresh Fruit (230 Calories)
- **Dinner**: Grilled Tofu with Steamed Broccoli (280 Calories)
- **Dessert**: Vanilla Protein Pudding with Cinnamon (150 Calories)
- **Total Calories**: 1040

Day 75
- **Breakfast**: Egg White Omelette with Spinach and Feta (180 Calories)
- **Lunch**: Shrimp and Avocado Salad (320 Calories)
- **Snack**: Overnight Chia Pudding with Almonds (200 Calories)
- **Dinner**: Turkey and Spinach Stuffed Peppers (280 Calories)
- **Dessert**: Almond Flour Chocolate Brownies (200 Calories)
- **Total Calories**: 1180

Day 76
- **Breakfast**: Cottage Cheese and Berry Smoothie (200 Calories)
- **Lunch**: Turkey Sausage and Egg Breakfast Burrito (250 Calories)
- **Snack**: Almond Butter and Banana Rice Cakes (245 Calories)
- **Dinner**: Baked Cod with Asparagus (300 Calories)
- **Dessert**: Berry Protein Smoothie Bowl (200 Calories)
- **Total Calories**: 1195

Day 77
- **Breakfast**: Scrambled Tofu with Vegetables (200 Calories)
- **Lunch**: Grilled Chicken Caesar Salad (300 Calories)
- **Snack**: Low-Fat Ricotta and Berry Toast (200 Calories)
- **Dinner**: Chicken and Zucchini Noodles (280 Calories)
- **Dessert**: Protein-Packed Chocolate Chip Cookies (175 Calories)
- **Total Calories**: 1155

Day 78
- **Breakfast**: Greek Yogurt Parfait with Berries (230 Calories)
- **Lunch**: Grilled Chicken and Veggie Wrap (320 Calories)
- **Snack**: Protein-Packed Chocolate Chip Cookies (200 Calories)
- **Dinner**: Grilled Lemon Herb Chicken with Zucchini Noodles (250 Calories)
- **Dessert**: Almond Flour Chocolate Brownies (200 Calories)
- **Total Calories**: 1200

Day 79
- **Breakfast**: Egg White Omelette with Spinach and Feta (180 Calories)
- **Lunch**: Tuna Salad Lettuce Wraps (200 Calories)
- **Snack**: Vanilla Protein Pudding with Cinnamon (200 Calories)
- **Dinner**: Grilled Shrimp with Cauliflower Rice (270 Calories)
- **Dessert**: Greek Yogurt Cheesecake with Fresh Berries (200 Calories)
- **Total Calories**: 1150

Day 80
- **Breakfast**: Protein-Packed Smoothie with Almond Milk and Berries (230 Calories)
- **Lunch**: Turkey and Hummus Roll-Ups (320 Calories)
- **Snack**: Low-Fat Ricotta and Lemon Tart (200 Calories)
- **Dinner**: Grilled Chicken with Zucchini Noodles (250 Calories)
- **Dessert**: Vanilla Protein Pudding with Cinnamon (200 Calories)
- **Total Calories**: 1200

Day 81
- **Breakfast**: Smoked Salmon and Avocado Toast (240 Calories)
- **Lunch**: Chicken and Quinoa Salad (320 Calories)
- **Snack**: Protein-Packed Chocolate Chip Cookies (200 Calories)
- **Dinner**: Grilled Salmon with Steamed Broccoli (290 Calories)
- **Dessert**: Greek Yogurt Cheesecake with Fresh Berries (200 Calories)
- **Total Calories**: 1250

Day 82
- **Breakfast**: Overnight Chia Pudding with Almonds (250 Calories)
- **Lunch**: Shrimp and Avocado Salad (300 Calories)
- **Snack**: Almond Flour Chocolate Brownies (200 Calories)
- **Dinner**: Turkey Meatballs with Spaghetti Squash (290 Calories)
- **Dessert**: High-Protein Chocolate Lava Cake (200 Calories)
- **Total Calories**: 1240

Day 83
- **Breakfast**: Turkey and Veggie Breakfast Wrap (250 Calories)
- **Lunch**: Turkey and Spinach Roll-Ups (320 Calories)
- **Snack**: Low-Fat Ricotta and Lemon Tart (200 Calories)
- **Dinner**: Grilled Shrimp with Veggie Stir-Fry (250 Calories)
- **Dessert**: Greek Yogurt Cheesecake with Fresh Berries (200 Calories)
- **Total Calories**: 1220

Day 84
- **Breakfast**: Low-Fat Greek Yogurt with Fresh Fruit (230 Calories)
- **Lunch**: Chicken and Black Bean Salad (345 Calories)
- **Snack**: Vanilla Protein Pudding with Cinnamon (200 Calories)
- **Dinner**: Grilled Salmon with Steamed Broccoli (290 Calories)
- **Dessert**: Almond Flour Chocolate Brownies (200 Calories)
- **Total Calories**: 1200

Day 85
- **Breakfast**: Greek Yogurt Parfait with Berries (230 Calories)
- **Lunch**: Grilled Chicken and Veggie Wrap (320 Calories)
- **Snack**: Blueberry Protein Muffins (180 Calories)
- **Dinner**: Grilled Lemon Herb Chicken with Zucchini Noodles (250 Calories)
- **Dessert**: Protein-Packed Chocolate Chip Cookies (200 Calories)
- **Total Calories**: 1180

Day 86
- **Breakfast**: Egg White Omelette with Spinach and Feta (180 Calories)
- **Lunch**: Tuna Salad Lettuce Wraps (200 Calories)
- **Snack**: Peanut Butter Protein Balls (180 Calories)
- **Dinner**: Grilled Shrimp with Cauliflower Rice (270 Calories)
- **Dessert**: High-Protein Chocolate Lava Cake (200 Calories)
- **Total Calories**: 1130

Day 87
- **Breakfast**: Protein-Packed Smoothie with Almond Milk and Berries (230 Calories)
- **Lunch**: Turkey and Hummus Roll-Ups (320 Calories)
- **Snack**: Protein-Packed Lemon Cheesecake Bites (180 Calories)
- **Dinner**: Grilled Chicken with Zucchini Noodles (250 Calories)
- **Dessert**: Vanilla Protein Pudding with Cinnamon (200 Calories)
- **Total Calories**: 1180

Day 88
- **Breakfast**: Smoked Salmon and Avocado Toast (240 Calories)
- **Lunch**: Chicken and Quinoa Salad (320 Calories)
- **Snack**: Low-Fat Ricotta and Berry Toast (200 Calories)
- **Dinner**: Grilled Salmon with Steamed Broccoli (290 Calories)
- **Dessert**: Greek Yogurt Cheesecake with Fresh Berries (200 Calories)
- **Total Calories**: 1250

Day 89
- **Breakfast**: Overnight Chia Pudding with Almonds (250 Calories)
- **Lunch**: Shrimp and Avocado Salad (300 Calories)
- **Snack**: Protein-Packed Chocolate Chip Cookies (200 Calories)
- **Dinner**: Turkey Meatballs with Spaghetti Squash (290 Calories)
- **Dessert**: High-Protein Chocolate Lava Cake (200 Calories)
- **Total Calories**: 1240

Day 90
- **Breakfast**: Turkey and Veggie Breakfast Wrap (250 Calories)
- **Lunch**: Turkey and Spinach Roll-Ups (320 Calories)
- **Snack**: Almond Flour Chocolate Brownies (200 Calories)
- **Dinner**: Grilled Shrimp with Veggie Stir-Fry (250 Calories)
- **Dessert**: Vanilla Protein Pudding with Cinnamon (200 Calories)
- **Total Calories**: 1220

Day 91
- **Breakfast**: Low-Fat Greek Yogurt with Fresh Fruit (230 Calories)
- **Lunch**: Chicken and Black Bean Salad (345 Calories)
- **Snack**: Peanut Butter Protein Balls (180 Calories)
- **Dinner**: Grilled Salmon with Asparagus (290 Calories)
- **Dessert**: Protein-Packed Chocolate Chip Cookies (200 Calories)
- **Total Calories**: 1245

Day 92
- **Breakfast**: Greek Yogurt Parfait with Berries (230 Calories)
- **Lunch**: Grilled Chicken and Veggie Wrap (320 Calories)
- **Snack**: Protein-Packed Lemon Cheesecake Bites (180 Calories)
- **Dinner**: Grilled Lemon Herb Chicken with Steamed Broccoli (250 Calories)
- **Dessert**: Vanilla Protein Pudding with Cinnamon (200 Calories)
- **Total Calories**: 1180

Day 93
- **Breakfast**: Scrambled Tofu with Vegetables (200 Calories)
- **Lunch**: Tuna Salad Lettuce Wraps (200 Calories)
- **Snack**: Cottage Cheese and Pineapple Delight (150 Calories)
- **Dinner**: Grilled Shrimp with Cauliflower Rice (270 Calories)
- **Dessert**: High-Protein Chocolate Lava Cake (200 Calories)
- **Total Calories**: 1120

Day 94
- **Breakfast**: Protein-Packed Smoothie with Almond Milk and Berries (230 Calories)
- **Lunch**: Turkey and Spinach Roll-Ups (320 Calories)
- **Snack**: Greek Yogurt with Cucumber and Herbs (120 Calories)
- **Dinner**: Grilled Salmon with Steamed Green Beans (290 Calories)
- **Dessert**: Low-Fat Ricotta and Lemon Tart (200 Calories)
- **Total Calories**: 1160

Day 95
- **Breakfast**: Smoked Salmon and Avocado Toast (240 Calories)
- **Lunch**: Chicken and Quinoa Salad (320 Calories)
- **Snack**: High-Protein Chocolate Mousse (160 Calories)
- **Dinner**: Turkey Meatballs with Spaghetti Squash (290 Calories)
- **Dessert**: Protein-Packed Chocolate Chip Cookies (200 Calories)
- **Total Calories**: 1210

Day 96
- **Breakfast**: Overnight Chia Pudding with Almonds (250 Calories)
- **Lunch**: Shrimp and Avocado Salad (300 Calories)
- **Snack**: Peanut Butter Protein Balls (180 Calories)
- **Dinner**: Grilled Chicken with Zucchini Noodles (250 Calories)
- **Dessert**: Almond Flour Chocolate Brownies (200 Calories)
- **Total Calories**: 1180

Day 97
- **Breakfast**: Egg White Omelette with Spinach and Feta (200 Calories)
- **Lunch**: Turkey and Hummus Roll-Ups (320 Calories)
- **Snack**: Greek Yogurt Cheesecake with Fresh Berries (200 Calories)
- **Dinner**: Grilled Lemon Herb Shrimp with Veggies (290 Calories)
- **Dessert**: Vanilla Protein Pudding with Cinnamon (200 Calories)
- **Total Calories**: 1210

Day 98
- **Breakfast**: Low-Fat Greek Yogurt with Fresh Fruit (230 Calories)
- **Lunch**: Chicken and Black Bean Salad (345 Calories)
- **Snack**: Cottage Cheese and Berry Bowl (150 Calories)
- **Dinner**: Grilled Salmon with Asparagus (290 Calories)
- **Dessert**: High-Protein Chocolate Lava Cake (200 Calories)
- **Total Calories**: 1195

Day 99
- **Breakfast**: Greek Yogurt Parfait with Berries (230 Calories)
- **Lunch**: Grilled Chicken and Veggie Wrap (320 Calories)
- **Snack**: Protein-Packed Lemon Cheesecake Bites (180 Calories)
- **Dinner**: Grilled Lemon Herb Chicken with Zucchini Noodles (250 Calories)
- **Dessert**: Greek Yogurt Cheesecake with Fresh Berries (200 Calories)
- **Total Calories**: 1180

Day 100
- **Breakfast**: Egg White Omelette with Spinach and Feta (180 Calories)
- **Lunch**: Tuna Salad Lettuce Wraps (200 Calories)
- **Snack**: Almond Flour Chocolate Brownies (200 Calories)
- **Dinner**: Grilled Shrimp with Cauliflower Rice (270 Calories)
- **Dessert**: Vanilla Protein Pudding with Cinnamon (200 Calories)
- **Total Calories**: 1150

Day 101
- **Breakfast**: Protein-Packed Smoothie with Almond Milk and Berries (230 Calories)
- **Lunch**: Turkey and Hummus Roll-Ups (320 Calories)
- **Snack**: Blueberry Protein Muffins (180 Calories)
- **Dinner**: Grilled Chicken and Zucchini Noodles (250 Calories)
- **Dessert**: Greek Yogurt Cheesecake with Fresh Berries (200 Calories)
- **Total Calories**: 1180

Day 102
- **Breakfast**: Smoked Salmon and Avocado Toast (240 Calories)
- **Lunch**: Chicken and Quinoa Salad (320 Calories)
- **Snack**: Protein-Packed Lemon Cheesecake Bites (180 Calories)
- **Dinner**: Grilled Salmon with Steamed Broccoli (290 Calories)
- **Dessert**: Vanilla Protein Pudding with Cinnamon (200 Calories)
- **Total Calories**: 1230

Day 103
- **Breakfast**: Overnight Chia Pudding with Almonds (250 Calories)
- **Lunch**: Shrimp and Avocado Salad (300 Calories)
- **Snack**: Almond Flour Chocolate Brownies (200 Calories)
- **Dinner**: Turkey Meatballs with Spaghetti Squash (290 Calories)
- **Dessert**: High-Protein Chocolate Lava Cake (200 Calories)
- **Total Calories**: 1240

Day 104
- **Breakfast**: Turkey and Veggie Breakfast Wrap (250 Calories)
- **Lunch**: Turkey and Spinach Roll-Ups (320 Calories)
- **Snack**: Protein-Packed Chocolate Chip Cookies (200 Calories)
- **Dinner**: Grilled Shrimp with Veggie Stir-Fry (250 Calories)
- **Dessert**: Almond Flour Chocolate Brownies (200 Calories)
- **Total Calories**: 1220

Day 105
- **Breakfast**: Low-Fat Greek Yogurt with Fresh Fruit (230 Calories)
- **Lunch**: Chicken and Black Bean Salad (345 Calories)
- **Snack**: Protein-Packed Chocolate Chip Cookies (200 Calories)
- **Dinner**: Grilled Salmon with Asparagus (290 Calories)
- **Dessert**: Greek Yogurt Cheesecake with Fresh Berries (200 Calories)
- **Total Calories**: 1260

Day 106
- **Breakfast**: Greek Yogurt Parfait with Berries (230 Calories)
- **Lunch**: Grilled Chicken and Veggie Wrap (320 Calories)
- **Snack**: Protein-Packed Peanut Butter Cookies (180 Calories)
- **Dinner**: Grilled Lemon Herb Chicken with Zucchini Noodles (250 Calories)
- **Dessert**: Greek Yogurt Cheesecake with Fresh Berries (200 Calories)
- **Total Calories**: 1180

Day 107
- **Breakfast**: Scrambled Tofu with Vegetables (200 Calories)
- **Lunch**: Tuna Salad Lettuce Wraps (200 Calories)
- **Snack**: Cottage Cheese and Pineapple Delight (150 Calories)
- **Dinner**: Grilled Shrimp with Cauliflower Rice (270 Calories)
- **Dessert**: High-Protein Chocolate Lava Cake (200 Calories)
- **Total Calories**: 1120

Day 108
- **Breakfast**: Protein-Packed Smoothie with Almond Milk and Berries (230 Calories)
- **Lunch**: Turkey and Spinach Roll-Ups (320 Calories)
- **Snack**: Greek Yogurt with Cucumber and Herbs (120 Calories)
- **Dinner**: Grilled Salmon with Steamed Green Beans (290 Calories)
- **Dessert**: Low-Fat Ricotta and Lemon Tart (200 Calories)
- **Total Calories**: 1160

Day 109
- **Breakfast**: Smoked Salmon and Avocado Toast (240 Calories)
- **Lunch**: Chicken and Quinoa Salad (320 Calories)
- **Snack**: High-Protein Chocolate Mousse (160 Calories)
- **Dinner**: Turkey Meatballs with Spaghetti Squash (290 Calories)
- **Dessert**: Protein-Packed Chocolate Chip Cookies (200 Calories)
- **Total Calories**: 1210

Day 110
- **Breakfast**: Overnight Chia Pudding with Almonds (250 Calories)
- **Lunch**: Shrimp and Avocado Salad (300 Calories)
- **Snack**: Peanut Butter Protein Balls (180 Calories)
- **Dinner**: Grilled Chicken with Zucchini Noodles (250 Calories)
- **Dessert**: Almond Flour Chocolate Brownies (200 Calories)
- **Total Calories**: 1180

Day 111
- **Breakfast**: Egg White Omelette with Spinach and Feta (200 Calories)
- **Lunch**: Turkey and Hummus Roll-Ups (320 Calories)
- **Snack**: Greek Yogurt Cheesecake with Fresh Berries (200 Calories)
- **Dinner**: Grilled Lemon Herb Shrimp with Veggies (290 Calories)
- **Dessert**: Vanilla Protein Pudding with Cinnamon (200 Calories)
- **Total Calories**: 1210

Day 112
- **Breakfast**: Low-Fat Greek Yogurt with Fresh Fruit (230 Calories)
- **Lunch**: Chicken and Black Bean Salad (345 Calories)
- **Snack**: Cottage Cheese and Berry Bowl (150 Calories)
- **Dinner**: Grilled Salmon with Asparagus (290 Calories)
- **Dessert**: High-Protein Chocolate Lava Cake (200 Calories)
- **Total Calories**: 1195

Day 113
- **Breakfast**: Greek Yogurt Parfait with Berries (230 Calories)
- **Lunch**: Grilled Chicken and Veggie Wrap (320 Calories)
- **Snack**: Protein-Packed Lemon Cheesecake Bites (180 Calories)
- **Dinner**: Grilled Lemon Herb Chicken with Steamed Green Beans (250 Calories)
- **Dessert**: High-Protein Chocolate Lava Cake (200 Calories)
- **Total Calories**: 1180

Day 114
- **Breakfast**: Egg White Omelette with Spinach and Feta (180 Calories)
- **Lunch**: Tuna Salad Lettuce Wraps (200 Calories)
- **Snack**: Almond Flour Protein Brownies (200 Calories)
- **Dinner**: Grilled Shrimp with Cauliflower Rice (270 Calories)
- **Dessert**: Vanilla Protein Pudding with Cinnamon (200 Calories)
- **Total Calories**: 1150

Day 115
- **Breakfast**: Protein-Packed Smoothie with Almond Milk and Berries (230 Calories)
- **Lunch**: Turkey and Hummus Roll-Ups (320 Calories)
- **Snack**: Low-Fat Ricotta and Berry Toast (200 Calories)
- **Dinner**: Grilled Chicken with Zucchini Noodles (250 Calories)
- **Dessert**: Greek Yogurt Cheesecake with Fresh Berries (200 Calories)
- **Total Calories**: 1200

Day 116
- **Breakfast**: Smoked Salmon and Avocado Toast (240 Calories)
- **Lunch**: Chicken and Quinoa Salad (320 Calories)
- **Snack**: Almond Flour Chocolate Brownies (200 Calories)
- **Dinner**: Grilled Salmon with Steamed Broccoli (290 Calories)
- **Dessert**: Protein-Packed Chocolate Chip Cookies (200 Calories)
- **Total Calories**: 1250

Day 117
- **Breakfast**: Overnight Chia Pudding with Almonds (250 Calories)
- **Lunch**: Shrimp and Avocado Salad (300 Calories)
- **Snack**: Protein-Packed Chocolate Chip Cookies (200 Calories)
- **Dinner**: Turkey Meatballs with Spaghetti Squash (290 Calories)
- **Dessert**: Vanilla Protein Pudding with Cinnamon (200 Calories)
- **Total Calories**: 1240

Day 118
- **Breakfast**: Turkey and Veggie Breakfast Wrap (250 Calories)
- **Lunch**: Turkey and Spinach Roll-Ups (320 Calories)
- **Snack**: Protein-Packed Lemon Cheesecake Bites (180 Calories)
- **Dinner**: Grilled Shrimp with Veggie Stir-Fry (250 Calories)
- **Dessert**: Almond Flour Chocolate Brownies (200 Calories)
- **Total Calories**: 1200

Day 119

- **Breakfast**: Low-Fat Greek Yogurt with Fresh Fruit (230 Calories)
- **Lunch**: Chicken and Black Bean Salad (345 Calories)
- **Snack**: Blueberry Protein Muffins (180 Calories)
- **Dinner**: Grilled Salmon with Asparagus (290 Calories)
- **Dessert**: High-Protein Chocolate Lava Cake (200 Calories)
- **Total Calories**: 1200

Day 120

- **Breakfast**: Greek Yogurt Parfait with Berries (230 Calories)
- **Lunch**: Grilled Chicken and Veggie Wrap (320 Calories)
- **Snack**: Protein-Packed Chocolate Chip Cookies (200 Calories)
- **Dinner**: Grilled Lemon Herb Chicken with Zucchini Noodles (250 Calories)
- **Dessert**: Vanilla Protein Pudding with Cinnamon (200 Calories)
- **Total Calories**: 1200

YOUR FREE GIFTS!

- **BONUS 1 - Survival Guide for Holidays and Special Occasions:** Learn how to enjoy parties and holiday treats without feeling guilty or compromising your health journey.
- **BONUS 2 - Wall Pilates for Women**: The easy-to-follow guide to supercharging your diet for incredible results.
- **BONUS 3 - Guided Mindfulness and Meditation Practices**: Discover how mindfulness can help you stay focused and stress-free on your weight loss journey.
- **BONUS 4 – My Weight Loss Journey:** Map your path to success with this printable plan and track your progress every step of the way.
- **BONUS 5 – Weekly Meal Planner**: Customize this printable meal planner and make your week of meals stress-free.

SCAN HERE TO DOWNLOAD

CONCLUSION

FINAL WORDS OF ENCOURAGEMENT

Embarking on a journey towards better health and weight loss can be challenging, yet immensely rewarding. Dr. Nowzaradan's 1200-Calorie Diet Plan is designed to guide you through this journey, offering a structured path towards achieving your health goals. It's normal to face hurdles along the way, but remember, persistence and dedication are key to success.

This diet plan is not just about losing weight; it's about embracing a healthier lifestyle that includes nutritious eating and regular physical activity. It's about making informed choices that benefit your body and mind. The recipes provided in this book, from the energizing breakfasts to the guilt-free desserts, are crafted to not only satisfy your taste buds but also to nourish your body.

Remember, every small step you take on this journey counts. Celebrate your progress, no matter how minor it may seem. Adjustments can be made, and it's okay to have days where things don't go as planned. What's important is getting back on track and keeping your eyes on the goal.

Your health and well-being are worth every effort. Stay committed, stay motivated, and let this diet plan be your companion in achieving the healthier, happier life you deserve.

STAYING COMMITTED TO HEALTH GOALS

Staying committed to your health goals is a journey that requires dedication, patience, and a positive mindset. It's about making consistent choices that align with your objectives, whether it's losing weight, improving your overall health, or both. Here are strategies to help you stay on track:

1. Set realistic and specific goals. Instead of aiming to "lose weight," target to lose a certain number of pounds within a specific timeframe. This makes your goals measurable and achievable.

2. Create a supportive environment. Surround yourself with people who encourage and support your health goals. This could be family members, friends, or a community of like-minded individuals.

3. Plan your meals. Use the recipes provided in this book to prepare healthy meals in advance. This helps prevent impulsive eating and ensures you stick to your diet plan.

4. Track your progress. Keep a journal of your food intake, exercise, and weight changes. Celebrating small victories can motivate you to keep going.

5. Be flexible. Life happens, and there will be times when you deviate from your plan. Instead of being hard on yourself, learn from the experience and get back on track.

6. Find activities you enjoy. Exercise doesn't have to be a chore. Discover physical activities that you look forward to doing, making it easier to incorporate them into your routine.

7. Manage stress. Stress can lead to emotional eating and derail your diet plans. Find healthy ways to cope with stress, such as meditation, reading, or taking a walk.

8. Stay hydrated. Drinking water can help control hunger and maintain your metabolism. Aim for at least 8 glasses a day.

9. Get enough sleep. Lack of sleep can affect your hunger hormones and lead to weight gain. Ensure you get 7-9 hours of quality sleep each night.

10. Seek professional help if needed. If you're struggling to meet your health goals, consider consulting a dietitian or a personal trainer for personalized advice and support.

Remember, the key to staying committed is not perfection but persistence. Every step you take towards your health goals, no matter how small, is a step in the right direction.

INDEX

Made in United States
Orlando, FL
08 January 2025

56994897R00054